I Love My Kids
But I Want
My Body Back

Dr Malcolm Linsell

Published in Australia in 2021 by Malcolm Linsell

Website: www.drmalcolmlinsell.com
Email: mlinsell4@gmail.com

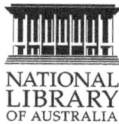

ISBN 9780648985006 (paperback)

A catalogue record for this book is available from the National Library of Australia

Photo credits
Front cover – Edwin Escobar (Urban Life Photography)
Jenny crossing the finishing line (p.118) – Marathon-photos.com
Author photo 1 – (in suit) Andy Taylor
Author photo 2 – (operating theatre) Mater Health

Disclaimer
The author has made every effort to ensure the accuracy of the information within this book was correct at the time of publication. The author does not assume and hereby disclaims any liability to any party for any loss, damage or disruption caused by errors or omissions, whether such errors or omissions result from accident, negligence, or any other cause.

To the thousands of patients who have trusted, and continue to trust, me with their faces and bodies. I am privileged beyond measure.

Ten per cent of profits from the sale of this book will be donated to Medicins Sans Frontieres (Doctors Without Borders) and Interplast Australia.

Contents

Foreword

When Dr Linsell told me he was writing a book about cosmetic surgery, I was excited. I have great respect for Dr Linsell and his excellent standard of work. But, more than that, he is truly empathetic with all who enter his clinics so I knew it would be worth reading.

I first met Dr Linsell some years ago when I was teaching a paramedical aesthetics course at a private hospital where he operated. He gave such a good speech to my students that they were talking about it for the rest of the course. When *Vogue Australia* started their beauty events (for which I was the MC), I straight away contacted Dr Linsell to ask him to talk about cosmetic surgery. I managed to get him to talk twice and, on both occasions, the attendees declared him not only the best and most interesting speaker, but they also felt that his patient before and after photographs were first rate.

I was lucky enough to get a first draft of his book and felt that this was indeed a book which women had been waiting for and, by the time I'd finished it, I was certain.

Every time I wrote a 'real person' cosmetic surgery story in *Vogue*, the readers loved them. So I know that the opportunity to really find out all of the details from a woman's first consultation, through to their reasons for surgery, and finishing up with the impact on their lives post-surgery, would prove to be so valuable to a reader's decision-making process. These interviews are real – warts and all. The wonderful women who told their stories do not hold back; they allow you to go through the whole journey with them.

I would absolutely ask you to read this book from cover to cover before you make a decision about cosmetic surgery. I feel so privileged to have been given the opportunity to get to read this wonderful book.

Ricky Allen *BSc BHSc. Dip.N. Dip.PA.*
Former Cosmetic Enhancement and Anti-Aging Editor for *Vogue Australia*

Introduction

I love to make a difference in people's lives. It's in my DNA. While my parents and grandparents felt called to make a difference through the church as Salvation Army Officers, I decided I wanted to be a doctor at the age of six. Almost 20 years later, my name was among those posted outside the Monash Medical School at the Alfred Hospital in Melbourne, Australia, confirming that a long-held dream had become a reality. It was one of the greatest days of my life. To be trusted with a person's intimate details about their health and for them to allow me to care for them by performing surgery is one of the greatest privileges I can imagine. Furthermore, most of my patients requesting cosmetic surgery are female and because, for a period of time, they have allowed me to be a part of their world, this book is written to honour them.

Women, particularly mothers, never cease to inspire me. Since I started plastic surgical practice nearly 30 years ago, I have worked with women almost every day. Sometimes they are challenging because they occasionally speak in a language that I (and most other men) were never taught. Remarkably, this language is understood by other women, who occasionally, if we men are genuinely interested, will take the time to translate and even extrapolate on what was said. Why is it that one woman can say a few words (or even not say anything) and a second woman can totally understand what the first woman meant, which may then take the second woman several minutes to explain?

Mostly, however, women simply amaze me. For instance, hospitals can be quite impersonal places at times. When a woman presents to hospital for cosmetic surgery, she has so many things on her mind. She has usually had to organise time off work, arrange for her children to be looked after, explain to her children why Mummy is out of action for a while, often pre-cook meals and make sure her husband or partner understands what is required for the next few weeks while her body heals. She has also been selective with which friends and family members she has told because she knows that not all of them will be supportive. Typically, all of that has been accomplished before she has even considered herself and how she feels. She is often terrified (for reasons we will discuss later) as she is confronted with one of the most vulnerable times of her life.

When she presents for surgery, it can be weeks or months since our consultation. On the day of the operation, I usually see her a few minutes before she is taken to the operating theatre. She is usually naked apart from a flimsy hospital gown that gapes at the back, she has no makeup or jewellery and may only be separated from the patient next door (who might be telling his nurse about the problems with his prostate) by a paper curtain.

I will ask her how she is feeling and invariably she will say something like, 'excited and nervous' which, if interpreted, would mean, 'I've never been so scared in all my life. I can't believe I'm letting you do this to me, and I trust you to do the very best job you can because I've gone through a lot to be here!'

The marking-up process is one of the most important parts of any cosmetic surgical operation. Any inaccuracy of measurements can contribute to a less than ideal result. Before I commence drawing on a patient's breasts or tummy, surely one of the most intimidating moments she will experience, I usually explain that this is a hospital and at any time anybody could burst through the curtain. Most mothers just laugh and say that they lost all dignity at the time they had their children, so it doesn't really matter who walks in. That is not really something a man would say. Women never cease to amaze me!

In the pages that follow you will meet several amazing women. They are heroes. They are the ones who had the courage to transform their bodies, and in so doing created for themselves more comfort, more choice and a boost in confidence that makes a difference in their lives and those who are around them. I have been privileged to work with these women to help them get their bodies back. They will explain what this has meant for them and what they went through in order to get there.

I have found their stories inspiring. I trust you will as well.

PART ONE

Why Have Cosmetic Surgery?

Why would a woman have cosmetic surgery? Because she can!

My mum had three children. I'm the eldest, then my brother Derek and the youngest is my sister Denise. Mum was 36 when Denise was born and, while I don't know for sure, I suspect she was left with the usual body changes that accompany pregnancy. However, as was typical in the 1960s, Mum simply accepted the changes to her body as part of being a mother and wore them proudly. Cosmetic surgery in the 60s wasn't a thing! Not that it didn't occur; it was just not socially acceptable.

When I commenced plastic surgical practice in 1991, not a great deal had changed. As part of my training, I had worked with, watched and assisted some excellent plastic surgeons performing cosmetic surgery, learning how to move my hands to create the best possible outcome in the least possible time. Cosmetic surgery was becoming more popular yet, as I look back, there was little finesse. Liposuction was in its infancy; the silicone within breast implants would leak if the implant was damaged; during a breast reduction, nipples were often removed then replaced as a skin graft; and tummy tucks would often tighten skin but do little to improve the shape.

Almost 30 years later, cosmetic surgery is now a 'thing' and has become socially acceptable. Gen Ys are leading this charge as young women in particular have no qualms with altering their appearance through either non-surgical or surgical means and I suspect this trend will only magnify as Gen Zs exert their influence. Meanwhile, nowadays the Baby Boomer generation has embraced cosmetic surgery as a real option, particularly for addressing some of the issues many women experience with their post-pregnancy bodies.

What has changed? There are numerous reasons attributed to the growth in cosmetic surgery but let's focus on five of the main ones.

1. Childbirth is occurring later in life

Women are having their children later in life. According to the Australian Institute of Health and Welfare, the average age of women who give birth has increased from 29.9 years in 2007 to 30.6 years in 2017. Furthermore, almost one in four mothers in Australia is aged 35 years when they have their first child.

2. Career first: Family second

The reasons women are having children later in life are numerous but one of the most common is that they are putting their careers first.

My wife, Kim, and I have two daughters, Rebekah and India. Both are 29, both beautiful and both highly educated. Rebekah has a Commerce degree, loves AFL and currently works for the Richmond Football Club. She will be a CEO one day.

India has a Bachelor of Medical Science and is currently studying dentistry. In a couple of years, she will finish her training with both a degree and a Masters of Dentistry, then take over her mother's successful dental practice in Sydney.

Neither woman is married, though one is in a long-term relationship. At this stage, one doesn't want to have children while the other is open, but a long way down the track. Both love the careers they have chosen and are fully focused on developing themselves to be the best business person and dentist they can be. It is career first. If a family happens, that's great but it is not a priority just now.

3. Financial independence

Rebekah and India are typical of well-educated Gen Y women. If, and when, a family happens, I do know that they will both have financial independence.

Both women are already financially astute and both women can expect to be earning above-average salaries in a few years. Gone are the days of my childhood when a husband earned the funds for the household and the stay-at-home mother needed to ask permission to use some of these for a personal purchase. Nowadays, young women are not reliant on their husbands or partners for their finances, giving them more choice over how household funds are used. If a woman chooses to have cosmetic surgery, somehow she will make sure she finds the funds so she can get access to what she wants.

4. Media

On a daily basis, women are bombarded with images and stories that directly or indirectly refer to the transformation of a woman's body. The increased awareness of cosmetic surgery has stemmed from exposure on our televisions, in magazines, in newspapers and on billboards to name a few. At the forefront is the explosion of social media led by celebrities and influencers demonstrating how their bodies can be transformed. Some admit to cosmetic surgery, some don't, but the effect is that, as one woman said to me, 'If Beyoncé or Kim Kardashian can look that good after childbirth, why can't I?' The rise of the selfie generation only perpetuates this because we all know that any time of the day (and night) our image can be snapped and uploaded, with or without our permission. If we are self-conscious about any part of our image, we either have to learn to put up with it or change that which is causing the distress.

The increased awareness of cosmetic surgery is a marketer's dream and has been seized upon by some, to promote the services of those who may not have the training or skills to consistently provide good outcomes for their patients. In Australia at the moment, a medical degree is called a Bachelor of Medicine and Bachelor of Surgery (MBBS). As undergraduates, we learn a little theory on surgery, but few medical graduates have performed any surgical procedures by the time they graduate. Unfortunately, under Australian law as it stands, any medical graduate can perform surgery, without any further surgical training. Hence the rise of the so-called 'cosmetic surgeon' who, in many instances, has had minimal surgical training and yet can advertise as a cosmetic surgeon who performs cosmetic surgery. This is in such direct contrast to fully trained and qualified plastic surgeons, who have had six to ten years formal training on top of their medical degree and then sit exams set by the Royal Australasian College of Surgeons. If they pass, they become Fellows of the Royal Australasian College of Surgeons (FRACS). If they don't, they need to sit again until they are good enough.

Australian plastic surgeons generally become members of the Australian Society of Plastic Surgeons (ASPS) and those interested in performing cosmetic surgery generally are accepted into membership of the Australasian Society of Aesthetic Plastic Surgeons (ASAPS). Both of these plastic surgical bodies hold us to account over what we do and how we interact with our patients. When you have surgery performed by a plastic surgeon with FRACS after their name and who belongs to ASPS and/or ASAPS, you know they have achieved a level of excellence with their craft, having been trained to be among the best in the world.

Buyer beware. If you have surgery performed by a cosmetic surgeon, either in Australia or overseas, you will probably get it cheaper (and may even have a holiday thrown in) but you increase your risk, particularly if something goes wrong.

5. Safety

Cosmetic surgery is real surgery. Real surgery has risks of complications which can range from: bleeding or infection, problems with healing, poor surgical outcomes, through to death arising from either an anaesthetic or surgical complication. For instance, a procedure commonly known as the Brazilian Butt Lift (BBL) has become a more sought-after procedure in recent years. It involves removing fat from one area of the body then transferring it to the buttock region to provide a larger, more rounded buttock. I have done this procedure a few times and both my patients and I have been pleased with the results. However, if the fat is injected into the buttock in a particular way, a bolus of fat can be injected directly into one of the large buttock veins. This bolus of fat (called a fat embolus) travels directly to the heart and the heart stops. In my view, too many healthy young women have died from this procedure and, consequently, I have stopped doing it altogether. The procedure would still be safe in an extremely experienced surgeon's hands but, around the world, these surgeons would be few and far between.

Nevertheless, improved anaesthetic and surgical techniques have made cosmetic surgery a much safer option than it has ever been. For instance, when I commenced practice, a women undergoing an abdominoplasty (tummy tuck) without liposuction, would normally be admitted to hospital the night before the operation, then stay in hospital for a minimum of three nights after the operation, unable to shower because of her bulky Elastoplast dressings, then go home, sometimes with her drains still attached. Nowadays, liposuction is usually included with an abdominoplasty, I don't use drains, there will be thin waterproof dressings so she can shower immediately and, in the vast majority of cases, she will go home the same day as the operation. Downtime and recovery have been dramatically reduced and, at the same time, patient acceptance has increased.

Cosmetic surgery can bring with it many advantages, yet it is still real surgery. With its commercialisation, many see it being the same as buying white goods from a retail store and, if something goes wrong, they can take it back and exchange it at no extra cost. It is not! Surgeons are not magicians and, though this may change in the future, you only have one body. If the surgical outcome is not ideal, a second procedure may be necessary, and this will cost you more money. The best time to get it right is the first time, and you increase your chances of this with a well-qualified, experienced surgeon who has taken the time to listen to your desired outcome and is confident of providing it for you.

Therefore, it helps to be cautious, to be well researched, to ask your general practitioner and/or friends for their recommendations. Even with all that, there is one important element that is required before contact is made with a plastic surgeon of your choice. That element is courage.

Courage

Any woman who makes an appointment then follows through with a consultation with a plastic surgeon, intending to alter a body part, is demonstrating an enormous amount of courage.

Unlike most forms of surgery, cosmetic surgery is a choice. No one has to have a facelift or a breast augmentation or an abdominoplasty or any of the cosmetic procedures offered. A woman is not going to die if she, as one of my patients described, continues to 'roll up her breasts like an empty sock and fold them into her bra'. Furthermore, apart from the face, most other areas of the body can be covered by good underwear or clothes and it is usually only a select one or two who might see her naked.

Nevertheless, a woman's quality of life can be deeply impacted by areas of her body she doesn't like. For instance, a woman with large breasts will suffer from constant backache, neck ache and shoulder ache. Normal activities such as running will be severely curtailed. From a young age she will find inter-actions with men to be different, for she will consistently find they will look at her chest, rather than her face. A woman with an abdominal overhang hates the feel of her tummy sitting on her lap. Some normal activities are also impacted for her and, in the summer, she is prone to sweat in the fold beneath the over-hang, leading to rashes and occasionally skin infection. Some women with small breasts, and particularly those with a flat chest, do not feel normal. They think they look like a boy and consequently do not feel feminine. To wear the clothes they want, they wear padded bras or use 'chicken-fillets' (silicone breast enhancers) to give the appearance they have breasts.

When a woman hates parts of her body, sexual intimacy can be a challenge because she will keep the part that she hates hidden from an intimate partner. She rarely feels free to relax because she is too self-conscious of the way she looks and/or feels about herself.

Feeling good about yourself has nothing to do with vanity. In my experience, vain people compare themselves with others, feeling they are better or superior. Most women I see want to feel normal, want to feel comfortable, want to be back to where they used to be. They have often tried non-surgical options with varying results but reach the point where, to make a lasting change and feel good about themselves, cosmetic surgery is an option and a choice they are willing to make.

For a mother, the choice comes with many considerations, as outlined below.

1. Terror

A mother is terrified she will die under anaesthetic. She is rarely concerned for herself; rather, she is concerned with the poten-tial disaster she feels she created in the first place. She feels she is choosing to put herself at risk, for something that doesn't need to be done, and if she dies, as one of my patients put it, 'How irresponsible is that!' She is thinking about who will look after the children, is it right for her to leave that responsibil-ity with their father or another family member, what it will be like for them to grow up without their mother and what will everybody think of her for choosing to have something done which she didn't really need?

2. Guilt

Consequently, she also feels that, perhaps for the first time in her life, she is putting herself first and she is feeling guilty, because she feels she is being selfish. Not only is she putting herself at risk, but she is spending money on herself when that money could be used for school fees, a family holiday, paying off the mortgage, a new car or a new motorbike for her partner.

Sometimes, during the consultation, if I get the sense these thoughts and feelings are bubbling under the surface, I will talk about them with her. If I do so, I know I need to have the tissues handy for invariably she will dissolve into tears when she knows that someone understands what she is going through.

3. Anxiety

Mixed in with the terror and guilt, she feels anxious about the choices she has made and is about to make. Is this the right procedure for her, has she chosen the right doctor, will he/she understand what she really wants and give her the best result possible and, most importantly, will she be cared for before, during and after the surgery? Many women are used to being in control, making decisions about the family and organising all the minute details that constitute family life. In this instance, to get what she wants, she is putting her trust in someone who has probably been recommended by others but, in spite of all the qualifications and supposed skill, he/she is still a stranger at a time when she feels most vulnerable.

4. Negative influences

Some or all of the above is going on in her own mind and heart and this is often before she has even talked to anybody else.

Even here she has to be very selective, because many well-meaning (and some not so well-meaning) family members and friends, just simply don't understand why she is making this choice and will try to talk her out of it.

Some are well-meaning but misguided. They have heard of a friend of a friend who had a disaster with her cosmetic surgical experience. This may or may not be factual, but it is a bit like telling someone not to drive a car because they know of a friend who had a car accident.

Others make out as if they are genuine but are actually jealous that she has the desire and the means to have cosmetic surgery. Relationships are challenging at any time and beware of the person who feels they are better than you, for whatever reason, and knows that if you follow through with surgery that reason will disappear. Furthermore, don't be surprised if some you considered to be friends before your surgery, break off the relationship with you after surgery. When it all boils down, the reason will be that they are jealous of you.

It astounds me that I have patients who were effectively blackmailed into cancelling their surgery because their children threatened to never forgive them if they proceeded.

On the other hand, nowadays I find most husbands or partners are supportive of their wife's decision. Invariably, the woman feels the most supported when her partner tells her that he loves her as she is, that she doesn't need to change, but if she wants to, she has his full support. It takes genuine love and a deal of courage for a man to say that because sometimes he might be thinking that his wife is going to 'fix herself up, then leave him for someone else'. I admire the man who accompanies his wife to the consultation, affirms his love for her, then stays silent unless asked by his wife for some input.

5. Fear of intimacy

Most of the above takes place in a woman's mind before she comes to be sitting in my consulting room. Experiencing the terror, guilt, anxiety and judgements of others, and still taking action to keep an appointment, takes an enormous amount of courage.

Yet here she is, describing to me (a person she only met a few minutes before) the areas of her body she hates and asking what can be done about them. To give a woman what she wants, it is important for me to be really clear about her ideal outcome. I will therefore draw her out a little, asking her how she wants her tummy or breasts to be and, more importantly, what clothes she doesn't wear now but wants to be able to wear in the future. There is a misconception, I suspect mostly from men, that women want cosmetic surgery so they will look good naked. I'm sorry guys but that is not their primary concern. They want to buy the clothes they like and know they look good in them. They want to wear tight-fitting clothes and no longer wear baggy outfits to cover what they perceive as their defects. They want the option to go without a bra, wear backless, strapless dresses, wear a bikini without padding or simply not have to think about the clothes they wear. If they look good naked, then that's a bonus!

Not only does she have to talk to me about what she perceives as her defects, she then has to show me. This is easier for some than others because they are essentially exposing what they consider to be the worst parts of themselves. She then lies exposed while I draw on her body, describing where incisions are made and the expected outcome.

I never take this for granted. I am aware of the courage it takes and am honoured that she trusts me enough to be exploring the possibility of correcting what she considers to be a defect.

Trust is the key. When she first made the appointment to see me, she already assumed I could give her what she wanted. She is now wanting to *believe* that I can. Moving from assumption to belief requires trust. She needs to know that I will always act in her best interests, that I won't abandon her, even if things go wrong. She needs to know that I care. My aim is to be open, authentic, honest and available. I will listen to her, asking her to describe her ideal outcome and, if I am confident I can provide this for her, I will repeat it back to her. Because I travel so much, she needs to know I am always available. Consequently, every patient has my mobile phone number and they know they have 24/7 access to me. Every patient knows they can contact me or send me photos at any time. I explain that I am used to receiving photographs of women's bodies at all hours of the day and night. My wife, Kim, is a dentist and she is used to it as well. When mothers know they will not be abandoned, before, during and after one of the biggest events of their lives, they feel reassured and in good hands.

PART TWO

In the following chapters, you will read the stories of several women who overcame their fears and doubts to follow through with surgery aimed at restoring their bodies back to where they used to be. They have had a variety of procedures on their breasts, tummies or faces, and sometimes procedures were combined in the one operation. These are all my patients who had their operations performed in Melbourne, Sydney, Cairns and Rockhampton. They come from all walks of life and my hope is that you will identify with them as normal women with the familiar challenges of motherhood and life in general.

I will describe a little of the technical side of what was done and they will share why they chose cosmetic surgery, what the experience was like and the impact it has had on them and those around them. Some of the stories have been written by me after interviewing the patients about their experiences. Some, the patients wrote themselves and have been reproduced with minor editing. Most names have been changed for privacy reasons.

To me, these women are heroes and their stories are inspiring. Their stories, and those of hundreds of others whom I have been fortunate to look after, are the reason I love what I do. To make a difference in a person's life is at the core of my being. To be trusted to be able to do this in this way is one of the greatest privileges I can imagine.

JANE – Tummy Tuck, Breast Augmentation and Lift

Early life

Jane was born in country northern Victoria into a very supportive family. Her parents separated when she was a teenager, but the family has remained close. She is the youngest of four children and, as both her parents worked full-time, she spent a lot of time on their small hobby farm without parental supervision. She became capable, confident and independent, resulting in good decision-making skills and maturity at an early age.

She enjoyed primary school, but not high school which she found irrelevant and she preferred to be out working in the supermarket after school, sometimes until late in the evening. She completed Year 12 then, with a few school friends, moved interstate, where after several hospitality jobs, she began an administration role with a recruitment firm. It was here she met her future husband.

The children

Jane has now been married seven years. She and her husband have three young children under six, one girl and two younger boys. Their youngest was a surprise. She discovered she was pregnant just days after her husband had accepted a promotion, requiring relocation to a city, thousands of kilometres away. They had no friends or family in the new city and the new role for her husband meant he was away from the house three to four nights per week. Nevertheless, they moved, and Jane chose to be a stay-at-home mum.

Effects on her body

After the birth of her third child, Jane struggled to get her body back to how it used to be. Her older sister, after four children, had the same trouble and while her sister was able to regain a reasonably flat tummy, her breasts were another story. Jane observed first-hand how this affected the way her sister felt about herself, particularly, when she separated from her partner. Jane noticed that her sister's confidence plummeted.

Jane's three children were born close together, which seemed to create greater havoc with her body. She felt that neither abdomen nor breasts came out the other side very graciously or functionally. She saw physiotherapists who said the wide separation of her abdominal muscles would come back if she would 'give it time'. Personal trainers on the other hand wouldn't work with her because of her abdominal separation. She felt the physiotherapists were just too keen to take her money, while the more research she did suggested that her separation was never coming back together. She felt she was doomed to look pregnant forever and feel uncomfortable in her own skin.

Prior to her children, her tummy was one of her greatest assets, always flat, but most importantly very strong. It wasn't until after children that she realised how much she needed her abdominal muscles. Consequently, her back was in constant agony, as it worked hard to compensate for the weakness in front of her tummy.

On the other hand, she didn't think her breasts were too bad. They seemed to fill a bra where they were mostly held up and covered. However, when she took the bra off, the effects of three years of breastfeeding were very obvious as her breasts were droopy and empty.

Effects on herself

Jane became very self-conscious, in fact, quite a recluse, rarely leaving the house unless absolutely necessary. She felt some comfort from being in a new city where she didn't know anybody, so she didn't have to worry about running into people she knew. She spent her time cooking and, on occasions, regretted having children as she was so unhappy, particularly when they were a little out of control. She felt present physically but absent mentally.

Jane's clothes reflected her mental state. She wore maternity or nursing clothes from when she was five months pregnant with her first child right through to after the birth of her last child. She felt sloppy and unattractive. Even when she attempted to dress up, her mind chatter reminded her of old sayings such as, 'You can't put lipstick on a pig'. One day a drunken family member said, 'You still have a pretty face' and someone else responded, 'Yeah, but you don't fuck a face'!

Considering cosmetic surgery

Jane's youngest was only 12 months old when she realised that her goal of getting her body back wasn't going to happen naturally. She had rolled her ankle early in the year and had seen a different physiotherapist. She briefly mentioned her abdomen to him to gauge his reaction and he laughed it off saying, 'That's never coming back'.

At the time, her mum was visiting and said that if cosmetic surgery had been an option after her children, without question, she would have done it. So, Jane and her mum began Googling and researching, just for fun at that stage. They mentioned it to Jane's husband at dinner, and surprisingly he was very supportive, though Jane expected some hesitation from him when he eventually found out how much it would cost.

She still wasn't sure if she would go ahead but kept researching. She joined forums, Facebook groups, watched videos, read many articles both for and against, and spoke to a close friend who had undergone breast augmentation. As part of her research, she discovered my name and was comforted by the fact she couldn't find a negative review, article or comment online. On a whim, she phoned and booked an appointment. She was expecting this process to be a little more difficult, but it seemed so easy. She still wasn't sure if she was going to follow through with surgery, but she and her husband decided to, 'Just see what he says'.

The consultation

Leading up to the consultation, Jane was very nervous, not sure what to expect. The last thing she wanted was some slick, arrogant surgeon who had an unrealistic expectation of mothers. Furthermore, after having three children, she was sick of having to undress for strangers, so she was not looking forward to it.

Yet, she describes feeling immediately comfortable and confident once we had met. She felt heard, understood.

Her ideal outcome was for her abdominal muscles to be together again so she could build on the strong foundation she once had. Her umbilical hernia could be repaired at the same time. She was more nervous about her breasts. Looking natural was very important to her so getting the right size was critical and in particular she did not want to look fake!

The procedures were discussed with her in detail, but she didn't want to take too much notice. She knew that some of the risks would keep her awake at night.

Nevertheless, as she walked away from the consultation, Jane knew that she wanted to have the procedures and she wanted me to do them for her.

Pre-surgery

From her research, Jane had a fair idea of the costs involved, so she wasn't surprised with the quote and neither was her husband, who remained supportive. She considered having just the tummy tuck alone but her husband and mother both felt it was best to have her tummy and breasts done together, because two long recoveries might put her off ever getting her breasts done.

Jane was a little hesitant to tell her father as she wasn't too sure what reaction she would get. Nevertheless, she found him to be extremely supportive, even making himself available to help out after the surgery.

She felt anxious about telling her sisters. One struggled with her weight and the other was desperate to have a breast augmentation, while neither of them were in a good financial position. Jane knew they would not see this as a vanity thing, but she was worried there might be some judgement about how much she was paying. She needn't have worried. Both were ecstatic for her and not once did she feel judged.

On the other hand, her in-laws were told she was having a hernia fixed. No one else knew.

This was deliberate for two reasons. Firstly, she didn't want people judging her for the money she was spending on herself for what they would assume to be purely aesthetic reasons. Secondly, she didn't want people to think she got her body purely through surgery and was therefore 'fake'. She knew that she was going to get back into exercise after the surgery and wanted people to see the dedication she put into her workouts along with her perseverance.

As the day of surgery drew near, Jane felt incredibly nervous and in 'full stress-out preparation/organisation mode'. She meal-prepped and planned for the full six weeks of expected recovery. She booked her family in to care for her children and arranged the family's travel needs. She made 'busy book' folders for the kids. She cleaned the house so that everything was spotless. She was doing anything to keep her busy and away from Google!

Day of surgery

When the day of surgery dawned, Jane was so scared, she felt sick. That morning, when dropping off her daughter at kindergarten, Jane hugged her tightly, thinking only of the worst-case scenario. She explained to her teachers that there would be family picking her daughter up for a few weeks and she just broke down and cried. She told them she was having surgery but didn't go into detail as she couldn't bear to tell anyone what she was about to knowingly put herself through. The teachers explained to her daughter that Mummy wasn't going to be around for a few days and that she needed lots of help for a while.

I saw Jane just before the surgery, reassuring her and asking if she had any last-minute questions. As I drew on her breasts and tummy, she was terrified and cried again.

She was calmer in the operating theatre, because she knew at this point there was no turning back. She doesn't like the feeling of being out of control so felt vulnerable, knowing there was nothing she could do or say while asleep, and knew she could only trust me and my team to give her the best possible outcome. Yet, she was ready, and deep down, she was excited that a new chapter was about to begin. Nevertheless, she held onto my hand very tightly as she drifted off to sleep!

The operation

Jane underwent a breast augmentation with a mastopexy (breast lift) using tear-drop shaped, textured silicone implants. This was followed by an abdominoplasty combined with liposculpture to her abdomen and hips. At the same time, her umbilical hernia was fixed. Theatre time was three hours.

Post-op

When she woke in the recovery room, Jane began asking for me because, as she said, 'wasn't I just holding his hand?' Then she realised she had some pain. Her chest felt heavy and she was nauseous. There were a few minutes of great discomfort, but the nurses acted quickly and she was made comfortable soon after.

The first night was a bit of a daze. She slept then woke for more pain killers then felt sick from the pain killers and repeat. This was unpleasant. However, it was just one night, and as every hour passed, she knew she was healing and becoming more mobile. She had known it was going to be tough, but it was perhaps a bit more so than she had hoped. It was the first night she had spent without her children in close to five years.

Initially it was only planned for her to stay in hospital one night, but she felt she wasn't ready to go just yet. In hindsight, she feels she should have organised two carers at home during the first week, one for the children and one for herself. Other patients have told me the same thing and it is a great idea.

The first week

The first week was a little harder than she was expecting. She had organised for her husband to be with her for the first two weeks, her mum for the following two weeks and her dad for the last two weeks. Having to rely on someone for assistance with simple everyday things distressed her and she felt quite vulnerable.

Looking back, she believes during the first night she may have strained something in her chest as she flinched while experiencing some nausea. Consequently, she believes her pain was worse than it should've been. She also had trepidations about the pain killers. Her husband had gone through a minor addiction to pain killers and she didn't want this to be her. Furthermore, she did not like the effect of the pain killers, which had her feeling so 'out of it' that she would again feel vulnerable. She had been so capable and independent for most of her life. Now, she really needed help and simply asking for some more water or assistance getting to the bathroom was something she was not comfortable with.

Jane called me on the phone, and I reassured her that many independent, capable women go through the same experience. Yet this was a time for her body to heal and she needed all the help she could get. She stopped the fight going on within herself, went for a check-up with the nurses, took all the pain killers she needed and found the courage to ask for help when needed.

This was easier said than done. Jane's husband had never managed the children on his own and she'd never asked him to help her with anything before. He was overwhelmed. He coped by going for walks when the children, and Jane, were sleeping. Early on there was tension in the relationship but as Jane became more mobile and less dependent, the tension eased.

The next few weeks

About three weeks post-op, Jane started to notice significant changes. Pain levels were still reasonably high for her, but manageable. Until that point, she hadn't really looked at herself. When her mum arrived, she began to help with grooming. The first thing Jane noticed was that she didn't look pregnant. She knew her breasts were still swollen, so she didn't pay too much attention to them at this point.

By four weeks post-surgery, Jane knew this was the best thing she could have ever done for herself. The pain was virtually gone. She felt very restricted with certain movements, but she was otherwise feeling great. Around this time, she noticed her abdominal wound had been rubbing on her support garment. This is not unusual because the wound is numb at this stage. It resulted in a small breakdown of the wound, but this healed quickly once she stopped the irritation of the garment. She also found she was allergic to the Micropore tape used once the original waterproof dressings were removed. Thereafter, rather than tape her wounds, she massaged them with Bio-oil on a daily basis.

By six weeks Jane started seeing the results she had wanted. Her confidence began to return. She was eager to start weight training and sculpt the body she had always wanted. Similarly, her husband began exercising regularly and eating healthily. He dropped weight and as they both began to feel good about themselves, their marriage became stronger and happier.

Back to normal

It took three to four months after her surgery for Jane to feel that she was back to normal. While she had felt very good at two months, she was still hesitant lifting and exercising. However, by four months she had started lifting weights and felt comfortable doing so.

By five months, she was super fit, lean and healthy, feeling happier with herself than she had been prior to having children.

Before and now

It is now more than 12 months since Jane had her surgery. Before her surgery she described herself as an unhappy, boring person. Now she loves exercising, looking after herself, and is much more active and confident. She has more fun and is more relaxed with life. Life no longer seems like a chore. Rather than just accepting things for the way they are, she feels that if something isn't the way she wants it, she has the power to change it.

Other people have commented on her physical changes, while a lot have also noticed how much happier she is now. Those who didn't know her before are astounded when they see photographs taken when she was pregnant.

Jane's husband is delighted. Both of them have been through significant changes and she now feels they are more attracted to each other than they have ever been. When she is naked, she is aware of the scars, though they are fading quickly. Yet, she is happy with what she sees. Before, she had been concerned her husband would be uncomfortable with the scars, but, typically, he doesn't even notice them.

Before, Jane felt that as a parent, she was very actively involved with her children. Now, she feels she has a much better relationship with them. She hasn't discussed it with them as they are still young, but she is now acutely aware of how a person's physical appearance can affect their life. When the time is right, it's a discussion she will have with them.

Clothes

Happily, Jane can wear anything she wants. She still needs to exercise, but she describes that freedom as wonderful. About five months post-op, she went to her favourite clothes shop while on holidays. The last time she had purchased from there was before children. The shop was busy and she felt a little old asking for help from the young sales assistants. However, within minutes they were picking out amazing outfits for her to try on, taking photos for their social media. Other customers also commented positively, asking to try on the outfits she had been modelling. In the change room, she had a quiet moment of reflection and shed a happy tear. She felt so proud, not only of her decision to have the surgery, but also to choose to be the best version of herself by continuing to strive to reach her fitness and health goals.

Advice to other women

While Jane doesn't tell people about her surgery, she identifies with a couple of friends who seem to be going through what she was going through pre-surgery. They've admitted to feeling depressed after looking at her, thinking she's one of those magical women who have got everything together after children. She's had a quiet word to them, told them what she's gone through along with all the ups and downs. She's told them it's the most terrifying and rewarding thing they could possibly do for themselves. She says, 'There's never a good time, now is the best time, why wait and be unhappy?'

Summing up

Jane says that, 'Life's good. I'm very happy with my decision. It's absolutely been worth it. It's the best thing I could have done for myself.'

Her one word to describe the whole experience … *'rewarding'*.

MALCOLM LINSELL

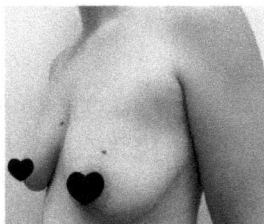
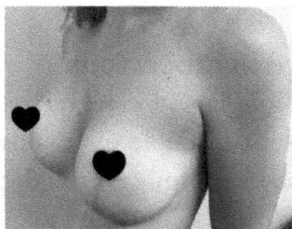
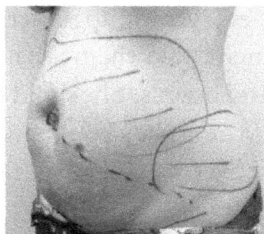
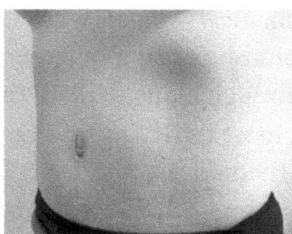

Before   *After*

JANE: Before and after TUMMY TUCK, BREAST AUGMENTATION and LIFT

CHELSEA – Breast Augmentation

Early life

Born in Central Queensland, Chelsea is the eldest child of three. She grew up on a cattle property, went to the local primary school, then boarding school 200 kilometres away. She describes herself as a typical country kid attending a public primary school and a private high school. She has worked as a station hand, legal secretary, bottle-shop attendant, waitress, bar attendant and, after completing her beauty therapy courses, now works as a self-employed beauty therapist as well as owning her own boutique.

Chelsea has been married to her soul mate for five and a half years and they have two children: a boy, five years old, and a girl, three years old

Effects on her body and self

With her pregnancies, Chelsea put on extra weight while her breasts lost most of the small volume she had as a young woman. She had been considering a breast enlargement since she was 15 but, with the birth of her second child, her confidence collapsed and she became critical of herself. Push up bras helped with the outward appearance but not with the inner thoughts.

Considering cosmetic surgery

Chelsea mentioned her struggles to a friend who had already had surgery, although things had not gone well for her. Her friend was supportive but because of her experience, urged Chelsea to do her research. This she did. She went online, browsing surgeons and their results, while continuing to talk with friends who had already had surgery. When she realised she was seriously considering doing this, she spoke with her husband. He was happy with her body as it was and had some concerns that an operation may not go well.

Chelsea wanted a surgeon she could trust and who had the experience to deal with any complications should they arise. Preferably, the surgeon would be local though she was prepared to travel if necessary. Chelsea was a friend of Mandy's, my executive assistant in Queensland so, by the time she had made an appointment to see me, she felt she was well researched and would be cared for should she decide to proceed.

The consultation

At the consultation, Chelsea was initially nervous but, because she had done some research, this helped to calm her. She told me that prior to children, she had worn a D-cup bra, which after two children had reduced to a B-cup. She had no plans for more children and would like to wear a DD-cup bra. Ideally, she would have more cleavage, be more in proportion and look natural both in a bikini and when naked.

I examined her, measured the size of her chest wall, drew where her scars would be placed, then took her photograph. Given her preferences, I felt a tear-drop shaped implant placed beneath the muscle would be the best option for her. She tried on a couple of implants of varying sizes and chose a 420 cc implant.

We then discussed the procedure in detail, going through what she could expect before, during and after the operation. We also discussed the potential complications in detail, outlining what we would do if any of them did happen to occur. Furthermore, I made her aware that I like to see every woman who has implants every 12 months for life, so we can be sure that all is well.

Pre-surgery

Chelsea left the consultation feeling excited. She felt heard and understood. As she had done her research, she knew what the costs would be and as she said, 'You get what you pay for'. This was something she wanted, she knew she could pay for it, and it was then a matter of arranging for someone to look after her children while she was recovering. She told her husband and a close friend because she knew they would support her. No one else needed to know. As the day of the operation drew closer, she felt nervous and excited.

Day of surgery

As the day of surgery dawned, she was nervous, worrying if it was the right decision to spend money on herself rather than her family. As she was being marked up, she became excited, then once in the operating theatre, as she was drifting off to sleep, she felt more reassured that this was right for her.

The operation

For Chelsea's breast augmentation, I used silicone tear-drop shaped, textured implants placed under her chest muscle. Theatre time was one hour.

Post-op

Chelsea's first night was uncomfortable. It often is with this operation because the muscle is stretched and this takes a week or so to settle. I saw her the next day and was happy with how she looked; however, for the first week, Chelsea was uncomfortable and worried that they weren't going to look very good. At home, she had a nanny to help with the children during the day and her husband to help in the evening.

It took a long time for Chelsea to be able to lift anything or look after the children without her new breasts hurting. It was four–five months before she felt back to normal, was able to go to the gym and perform her normal activities without discomfort.

Before and now

It is now 12 months since Chelsea's surgery. She likes her breasts, both clothed and naked. So does her husband. He said that, if he had known they would look so good, he would have encouraged her to have them done earlier. Her style of clothes hasn't changed a great deal; however, she enjoys showing off her cleavage sometimes in a tight or low-cut top, or bikini.

She feels more comfortable and confident, happy that she achieved the outcome she wanted and that the experience was not a waste of money.

Chelsea has also begun studying hairdressing which, at times, can be an intimidating industry. The confidence she has achieved since her operation has made a big difference here as she finds she has the courage to make decisions she might not have made before. This is something her husband has noticed and he has commented how he finds her courageous and inspiring.

Advice to other women

Chelsea advises other women to do their research and, as she found the recovery process to be quite painful, only go through with it if they are absolutely certain it is what they want. A good support network is imperative, particularly if you have small children.

She found that some chiropractic and massage work really helped to stretch her muscle to accommodate the implants and help her posture. Once healed, she also recommends daily stretches to help with any back discomfort.

Finally, bigger isn't always better. Chelsea was initially considering a larger implant (475 cc) before she chose the 420 cc size. Early after the procedure she doubted her choice and felt she could have gone bigger. Now she loves her size because they are in proportion with the rest of her body and are slightly easier to manage with work, movement and the clothes she wears.

Summing up

Chelsea knew what she wanted, had done her research, and demonstrated a lot of courage to follow through after hearing about her friend's poor experience with her breast implant operation. She found the recovery period a little more uncomfortable than most, but she has achieved the outcome she wanted, with no complications.

She is more comfortable, has more choice with the clothes she wears and feels more confident.

Her one word to describe her overall experience ... *'professional'*.

MALCOLM LINSELL

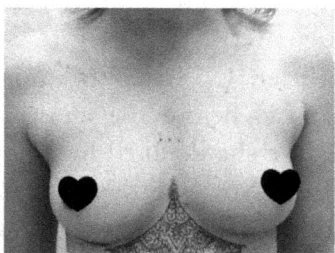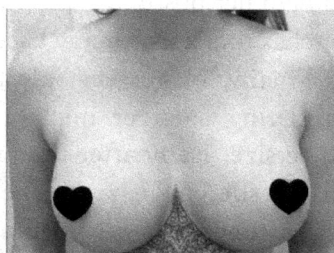

Before   *After*

CHELSEA: *Before and after BREAST AUGMENTATION*

JULIA – Implant Exchange, Mastopexy and Abdominoplasty

Julia has written her own story which is reproduced below with only minor editing.

Early life

I was a short and chubby child but blissfully unaware of both. My family immigrated from the UK when I was six. We lived in suburban Sydney and many of our friends were Scottish and English. I remember my parents' friends saying things like, 'If she's ever sick, she's got some meat on her to get her through' or 'She's a pretty girl, it's a shame; she's so bonnie'. I'm not sure it bothered me that much but I remember it all these years later and, most days of the week, I can't remember where I leave my keys or my phone so perhaps it did impact me more than I think. As a child, I was bookish and shy and had little interest in fashion or beauty or sport. I was the one who never got picked for any side for softball. I kind of lived in my own world and just loved my books and schoolwork. I came last in pretty much every sport but didn't really care as long as I remained an A student.

When I was around the age of twelve, we were all measured and weighed at school. I turned out to be the shortest person in my whole year but weighed more than my taller peers. That day I become aware of my body and it changed my whole mindset. I was already a driven child in terms of school – up early, studying always. When I realised I was basically short and fat, my natural drive and desire to do well kicked in. I didn't want to be that girl. I put myself on some weird and extremely unhealthy low-carb diet. I think it was called the 'army diet'. I tried all the fad diets, drank that foul and controversial Bai Lin tea, and started exercising every day. I gradually lost the weight. I preferred a strong, slimmer body and it opened a new world to me of being fit and eating well. By the time I was fourteen, boys started to notice me for the first time ever. Before that, I had been invisible and actually thought that boys would never be interested in me. I became interested in nutrition and fitness and I was so fearful of becoming the fat girl again, I probably got close to having an eating disorder. I struggled to go back to normal eating but, somehow, with the love of my parents and a good doctor, I didn't fall into the dreadful abyss of a full eating disorder.

From my teenage years right through to my 30s, when I started having kids, I was healthy and happy in my body. I remained a constant weight except for when I had break-ups with boyfriends. Stress has always impacted my appetite and I can't eat when I'm overly upset. I used to shed a few kilos after every break-up. In fact, I used to measure how heartbroken I was by how much weight I lost! The quicker I got over them, the quicker my appetite came back. Oh, those tumultuous years of dating. I thought they were hard enough but marriage was not much easier. But more thoughts on that later.

I kept exercising and, from those teenage years on, I have pretty much exercised every day of my life. For me, it keeps me strong and healthy and that always significantly impacts my mind and happiness. Just like I prefer to live in a modern, nice home, I also want to live in a strong and fit body.

Marriage and children

My journey into parenthood started with getting married. I met my former husband on holiday with friends in Spain. I was 34 and while I was in no hurry to get married, it was certainly something I wanted. He was Canadian, wickedly smart and funny, and sang like an angel. We fell in love and subsequently married.

My husband wanted children but I wasn't convinced. It was not because I felt they may interfere with my life and career. Rather, I knew that having a child meant that for the rest of my life, my happiness was entwined with theirs. There's a saying that you are only ever as happy as your unhappiest child. This scared me then and I now know it to be true. Having kids is the ultimate leap of faith because you are betting that they are going to turn out okay.

Whenever I am unsure of anything in life, I find it's because I don't have enough information and need to gather more. Being ambiguous about having children, I decided to research with my friends in order to understand their reasons for having children. Most of the answers I received were fairly simple, such as they'd been married for a few years and it was time, or they'd bought a new house and were ready to fill it with kids, or they were in their mid-30s and the clock was ticking. These answers didn't give me any faith. It was my dad and my Italian teacher, Roberto (an anthropologist, a professor and one of the wisest men I've met) who gave me a reason why. He told me that it gives your life purpose and makes you immortal. Not only are our children our flesh and blood, but everything we have learned we pass on to them.

So, with my new insights into having children, my husband and I embarked on the journey to become parents. When I'm on a mission, I'm on a mission and this time it was to get pregnant. It was all about measuring temperatures to find the right time and having my husband ready for on-demand and kind of clinical sex. It took about nine months, but I remember seeing those two lines on the pregnancy test and it was one of the best days of my life. I had always trusted that my body would know what to do and opted for a natural birth in hospital. I wanted no drugs at all. It turns out that my body had no idea about what it had to do! After about 14 hours, I asked for an epidural. I was on the verge of jumping out the window if I didn't get drugs fast. The pain! After 24 hours of labour, I was only 6 cm dilated, and the baby was getting very distressed. I needed to have an emergency caesarean section but didn't care as, afterwards, I had my beautiful baby boy. I exploded with a love like I had never known before.

I didn't have time to worry about recovery or getting my body back because, by the time my first son was three months old, I was pregnant again. Don't believe anything you hear about not getting pregnant while breastfeeding! Consequently, I had two baby boys in just over 12 months. Despite having easy children, those years were gruelling at times. I was back at work within four to six months after each child, albeit on reduced days per week. I was also exercising most days (thank goodness for the creche at the gym). It took over a year to get back in shape. Breastfeeding made me so hungry and it was very hard to diet. I remember still being about eight kilos over my usual weight and looking in the mirror wondering if I would ever wear a bikini again.

But healthy eating and exercise eventually worked. I got back to my normal weight, albeit with breasts that resembled empty cow udders and a stomach that permanently looked like I was about five months pregnant. The tummy improved but the boobs didn't. With the help of a push-up bra, I just learned to live with it and sought to be happy enough with the body I lived in.

Five years after my first child, much to my surprise as I had already hit 40, I fell pregnant with my third child – a girl. This time, after a pretty scary time with the first two births, I opted for an elective caesarean section. This was a breeze compared to my previous experience of emergency caesarean sections where, without medical intervention, both the babies and I would have died. Our bodies don't always know what to do!

So, there I was, a mother of three. Recovery from my third pregnancy never really happened. Sure, I lost the weight, but this was largely due to the breakdown of my marriage, subsequent sale of the house, and all the other challenges that break-ups bring. However, my breasts and stomach – in fact my whole mid-section – was not something that should ever be seen in public. I would do 200 sit-ups a day, a five-minute plank and more, and nothing ever changed. I still looked pregnant every single day, especially after I had eaten.

I've always been happy with my sexuality with few hangs up (at least I think I have). But I think the whole saggy, wrinkled, droopy mid-section influenced my intimate life. Honestly, looking down at my breast and belly if I were ever on top of my partner, would freak me out. It was like this body was not mine. Unfortunately, it was. If I were naked with my partner, I would be conscious of my body, always wearing a loose tee-shirt or putting my arms across my breasts when walking around. My partner wasn't bothered but I was.

Although I got used to it, I did everything in my power to make my body as fit as it could be. I wasn't obsessed, but every day I was conscious of how my stomach and breasts looked, and I dressed accordingly. Loose tops; loose dresses; trying to remember to hold my stomach in; always taking a side glance in the mirror when I went out to check I didn't look pregnant.

Considering cosmetic surgery

I didn't really think about getting it all fixed until I was on holiday with my friend Sarah, who happens to be a nutritionist and fitness guru. I was walking around the house in just bikini bottoms. I complained about my breasts and asked if there was any other exercise she could recommend for my ever-protruding stomach. Even after five years of my abs routine, I could still pass as pregnant. She tested my abs by getting me to lie on the floor and lift my head so she could feel if there was any separation in my muscles. Basically, I could put my entire fist between my stomach muscles which meant I had quite severe muscle separation. I learned later that I had an umbilical hernia as well. All this damage was from having children and could not be repaired by any diet or doing sit-ups all day long. Surgery was the only option.

So that's where it all started. I thought cosmetic surgery was for models and reality stars, not something for me. But I decided to investigate it as I always like to find solutions to problems.

I asked around, did research online, talked to my GP and interviewed three surgeons. Dr Malcolm Linsell was first. After my meeting with him, I didn't feel any need to see anyone else, but I did anyway, as gathering information for big decisions is always a good thing.

The consultation

Malcolm was warm and engaging. He listened and cared. He was patient with my indecisiveness. I met him a few times and we considered doing stomach or breasts or both. The cost brought many feelings of guilt, for I would be spending so much on myself. I could afford it because I would just take it out of the mortgage but, as a single parent, the cost seemed high. I felt guilty, terribly vain, and I struggled to reconcile the whole thing with myself.

Nevertheless, I decided to go ahead and do my breasts first as I wasn't sure if I would ever do my stomach anyway. Once I decided, I booked it in as soon as I could.

Day of surgery

I felt nervous and excited on the day. There was a little guilt as I considered I might die under anaesthetic. I knew the stats were so low that I probably had more chance of dying in a car accident. However, just in case, I rewrote my will and I wrote a letter to my kids.

The operation (*written by Malcolm*)

Julia had undergone a breast augmentation 16 years previously, so I accessed her implants through her original scar and found her left one was ruptured. Both implants were replaced with slightly smaller, round, textured, silicone implants. I then performed a breast lift. Theatre time was 90 minutes.

Post-op (*written by Julia*)

And before I knew it, it was all over. I was awake and in the recovery room, and Dr Linsell came in smiling, telling me all went well. I was in a surgical bra with underlying padding so I couldn't see anything.

I came out of hospital the same day. I preferred to be at home where I could eat my own food rather than hospital food, and sleep in my own bed. The pain was okay. I only took pain-killers for 24 hours and then just needed a sleeping pill to sleep at night.

I was desperate for a peek at my new breasts but refrained from looking for another 24 hours when I was ready to shower. Finally, I got to see them and, though bruised and swollen, they were fabulous. In fact, better than my breasts were before kids. They looked like they were the perfect size and shape for my body. Malcolm's recommendation was spot on. He's the expert so I trusted him to just pick the right model of implants for me.

I was back at work within days and life went back to normal. My boobs softened and the bruises went. I felt great and happy that they were fixed, and my body almost looked like it should do.

Two years later

Two years went by and my stomach still impacted my life. Every day I was conscious of it and found it affected my confidence in my body. Furthermore, since having children, I had suffered considerable back pain and learned that having my core repaired could assist with it. Knowing how much my breast surgery had impacted me, I decided to investigate the stomach surgery again.

One of the real concerns I had was being left with a large scar. I had healed well from all three C-sections but did have a large roll of unattractive fat or skin sitting above the scar. I was worried that the scar for a tummy tuck would be longer than a C-section scar.

Malcolm was always my trusted advisor. He never pushed me but gave me all the information and care I needed, then let me decide. I decided to proceed with a tummy tuck.

Day of surgery

And the day for surgery came again. I knew this was much bigger surgery and would take a couple of hours. Another will, another letter to my children, and a call to my boyfriend before I went under.

The second operation (*written by Malcolm*)

The separated abdominal muscle was repaired as well as Julia's umbilical hernia. Her excess abdominal skin was removed, and the area reshaped using liposuction. Theatre time was two hours.

Post-op (*written by Julia*)

Once again, I woke up to Malcolm's smile and reassurance that all had gone well. I decided to go home and not stay overnight for all the same reasons. This time, the pain was pretty intense. I needed a full week off work and my parents looked after my children for the week. I only took pain killers for 36 hours as I don't like the side effects, but I did need a sleeping pill to help with sleep. I was up walking my six kilometre walk in a few days, though I was quite slow. After a week, I was feeling pretty good.

And, oh wow, the difference was incredible. And my back pain was gone. It was one of the best things I have done for myself.

Before and now

I no longer dress to hide my stomach. Two years on, not only is the scar area completely flat, it's so faint I can wear a low-cut bikini and it's barely visible. Dr Linsell removed the C-section scars and left me with one super thin, pale and flat scar which is 100 times better than what I had before.

Sure, I am still ageing and getting crow's feet and all of that. But my body, which houses my mind and soul, and takes me through every challenge in life, is probably the best it can be at my age. I feel strong. I feel confident.

My partner also loves my repaired body and I'm far less self-conscious, which is good for our romantic life.

And the cost, which was probably the biggest hurdle for me? Well, I have never thought about it again. It's funny; our homes get wear and tear, and we have no hesitation renovating a bathroom or kitchen. Yet we 'borrow' our homes as they are rarely ours forever. But our bodies are forever so why not maintain and repair them too, particularly after having children?

My dear friend Ali, who is the same age and had the same surgery as me, has terminal cancer. Now that she is faced with her mortality, when I asked her if she regrets the surgery, as it all seems quite superficial now, she says, 'No way.' She wishes she'd had more done!

Advice to other women

Life can be short. Be the best you can be. Try to love the body you live in. Maintain and repair it so it lasts the distance.

Final thoughts

I was never a maternal person. It's always baffled me, that as little girls, we are quite maternal. We play with dolls, walk them in strollers, bathe them, and practise being mothers. Then, that instinct disappears and for me it never came back. I've ended up with three children and am a single parent who has my kids 100 per cent of the time, so life certainly did not quite turn out as I was expecting. I wasn't sure that I even wanted children, let alone raising three on my own. But they are the love of my life and I certainly have no regrets.

To be honest, I am not sure I am the marrying kind anyway. Despite growing up in a traditional household where my mum was the family caretaker and my dad, an accountant, the bread-winner who made all the decisions, I have always seen myself as an equal to men. I tried the good, supportive 'your career comes first' role, 'you manage the finances' etc. when I was married and I was bad at it. Now I am a big supporter of women and whatever choices they make. I have many friends in great marriages who gave up their careers and that works for them. For me, I've always thought having my own career and being able to make a reasonable living was empowering. I always needed to be more than a wife and mother, and contribute to the world in other ways, particularly in my work.

Nevertheless, I've willingly and happily given my body and decades of my life to raising children. I'm constantly trying to share wisdom and life lessons with my kids, especially now two of them are teenagers. I am not sure if they listen, but occasionally they surprise me, and I see the philosophies I've learned through life experience (and often bad decisions) have been instilled in them. I hope to live to be very old. But if I don't, I will leave feeling I contributed three wonderful human beings to the world and it will be their turn to inherit the earth.

They are a gift I don't take for granted. But I need to give back to myself too and this was my gift to me.

MALCOLM LINSELL

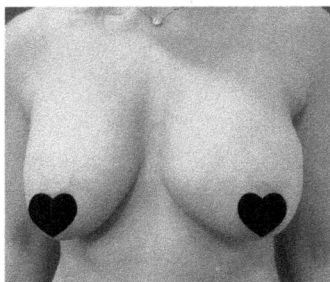 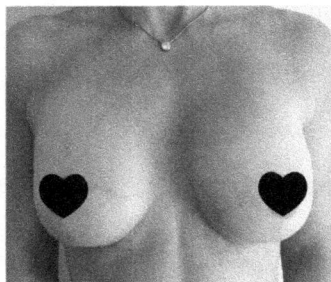

Before   *After*

***JULIA:** Before and after IMPLANT EXCHANGE and MASTOPEXY*

MALCOLM LINSELL

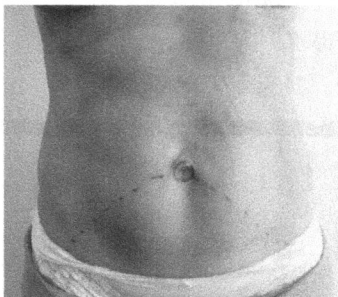
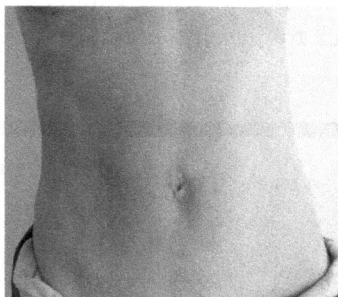

Before *After*

JULIA: Before and after ABDOMINOPLASTY

RACHEL – Breast Augmentation, Removal of Implants and Breast Lift

Early life

Rachel is the eldest of five children, born in one of Melbourne's satellite cities, in country Victoria. She attended the local Catholic primary school, followed by the public high school. Her childhood was active as all five children loved the outdoors so camping and fishing were a highlight, along with sporting activities such as basketball and netball. She recalls her mum and dad always saying, 'Go outside and play'. So, she and her siblings did – building cubby houses, riding bikes and making their own fun.

While still at school, Rachel commenced working part-time as soon as she was legally able, working 10 hours a week in the deli at the local supermarket. After completing her high school education, she went straight into the workforce and began an office administration traineeship. After several years, she commenced work at a registered training organisation as a workplace trainer and assessor. At the age of 35, Rachel returned to study at university as a mature-age student, study-ing a Bachelor of Early Childhood and Primary School.

Marriage and children

Many years ago, when Rachel met the man who was to become her husband, she knew that he was going to be the man that she would marry one day. She was right. They have been together 17 years and have now celebrated their 10-year wedding anniversary. They always support each other and she couldn't imagine her life without him. Together they commenced their own plumbing business and civil business; her husband does the plumbing and she does the bookwork in addition to her full-time job or study.

Together they have three children under nine years of age.

Effects on her body and self

Rachel grew up having large breasts; however, after having children, they became empty and saggy. Her weight had fluctuated throughout each pregnancy but after her final child, she lost her pregnancy weight and was fit and healthy.

Nevertheless, she found herself covering up her breasts to hide her insecurities. Wearing a pushup bra didn't help and she felt uncomfortable in swimwear. Her lack of confidence flowed over into the bedroom where she preferred the lights out when she was intimate with her husband.

Considering cosmetic surgery

Rachel had always joked how one day she would love to have breast implants, but never thought that it could happen. She didn't think she could ever afford it as they had three children and she felt surgery was a luxury, not a necessity. One of the times she joked about it with her husband he said, 'Well, why don't you get them done then?' She looked at him and said, 'Are you serious?' and he said, 'Yes I am. If it is something that is going to bring your confidence back, then it's going to be worth it, no matter the cost.' He continued, 'I will love you whether you have implants or not, but if it is something that is important to you, then I will support you, whichever choice you make.'

Being from a country town, she didn't want anyone to know what she was doing and went online to research her options in Melbourne. It was her gut feeling that led her to the practice where I was at the time.

Making the appointment was terrifying for her. She was totally out of her comfort zone, shaking and struggling to get her words out properly. She felt like a country girl going to the big smoke and when she was waiting in reception, she wondered if she had made the right choice.

The consultation

Rachel's recollection of the consultation is described best in her own words.

'I remember Dr Linsell walking out to reception and saying my name to go through to his room. That is when it hit me, this is happening. My heart was racing knowing that I had to take my top off to show him my most vulnerable part of my body. I clearly remember that not once did he look at my breasts, even when I had my clothes on, until I was standing there half naked. Dr Linsell made me feel at ease and comfortable, and it was then that I knew there was no need to visit any other surgeons for a second opinion. I am a believer of following your gut instinct and I am glad that I did. Dr Linsell drew all over me with a Texta and showed me the various types of implants should I choose to go ahead with the surgery. Not once did Dr Linsell put pressure on me to have implants and I feel this is such an important part of the process. Consequently, this life-changing decision was left 100 per cent up to me and me only.'

Rachel was able to describe her ideal outcome for me. She wanted to feel like she had her pre-pregnancy breasts again and not hanging down near her belly button. (They didn't actually hang that low, but to Rachel, they were on their way down there.)

She was given a copy of the information we had discussed and, as usual, I gave Rachel my mobile number and encouraged her to call, SMS or email me if she had any questions. She walked out and called her husband straight away saying, 'Yes, I am doing this'. She felt comfortable and was eager to book in a date for surgery as soon as she could.

Pre-surgery

Rachel knew the procedure would be costly; however, she thought, *You get what you pay for.* Her husband wasn't concerned with how much it was going to be as all he wanted was to see his wife full of confidence again.

Rachel asked her mum and sister to look after her children when she had the procedure and they were the only people she told. She didn't want to explain to people why she was having surgery and possibly be talked out of it.

She was ready, excited and counting down the days.

Day of surgery

When she was about to walk out the back door to head off to Melbourne for surgery, Rachel broke down in tears. Her husband asked what was wrong. Amidst the sobs, she expressed how she felt so overwhelmed and extremely guilty for spending all this money on herself, instead of on the children or saving to build their dream home. He gave her a hug and said, 'You need to put yourself first sometimes and it's going to be okay.' After the tears she smiled and realised her dream was actually turning into reality. She felt excited again.

When I saw her to do the marking up, she was still excited but, as with most people, a little nervous. I held her hand as she drifted off to sleep.

The operation

Rachel had a breast augmentation using high-profile silicone tear-drop shaped, textured implants placed under her chest muscle. Theatre time was one hour.

Post-op

When she woke, the first thing she remembers was wondering what her new breasts looked like. She had chosen to stay overnight in hospital and was sharing a room with a woman who had just gone through the same procedure. She found it enjoyable to talk with someone who had just been through the same process and hear her experiences. Prior to surgery, she had not known anyone who had been through the procedure and, in retrospect, would have loved to have been able to ask someone some questions.

The first weeks

Having young children at home was a challenge but her husband was fantastic. He helped with dinner and housework so that she could rest on the couch, keeping up with the pain killers and taking it easy.

Rachel knew it had all been worth it when she saw her breasts for the first time after surgery. She was so glad that she had done it. Then, at six weeks, when she wore a fitted bra for the first time, she was so happy. She kept looking at herself in the mirror to make sure it wasn't a dream.

Back to normal

It was two to three months before Rachel felt entirely back to normal. Her confidence was back, and she felt more like a woman again. Consequently, feeling like herself again, in the bedroom, she was happy to have the lights back on. Happy wife, happy life!

Before and now

It is the restoration of confidence that has made such a difference, so much so, that Rachel feels it is the best decision she has ever made. Her husband was happy before and after surgery. He didn't mind either way but just wanted her to be happy again. Her lack of confidence affected everyone around her, so when she was in a happier place, her family was happier.

She now feels comfortable to wear whatever clothes she feels like. Similarly, she is happy to be naked and is no longer covering various parts of her body. This was the outcome she wanted and feels it has been totally worth it.

Advice to other women

Rachel understands the guilt that comes with putting yourself first. However, she feels you need to do things for yourself in order to look after those around you. Then, if you have ever wanted to have surgery, go for it. Do your research and find a surgeon that you feel 100 per cent comfortable with.

Summing up

Rachel is so glad she went through with her surgery as it has changed her life and she has no regrets. One word to describe her experience … 'life-changing!'

Yet, Rachel's story doesn't end there.

As a routine, I see my patients who have had breast implants every 12 months for a check-up. Over the last few years, there has been some concern with an association between textured breast implants and a *rare* form of lymphoma, known as Anaplastic Large Cell Lymphoma (ALCL). There is a great deal of research underway to identify the causes of ALCL and at the time of writing it seems to be more commonly linked with implants that have a 'rougher' texture than others.

The most common presentation of ALCL occurs seven to ten years after the initial surgery, when the woman notices one breast becoming larger than the other. This is due to fluid accumulating around the implant and, if this occurs, an ultrasound is performed, the fluid drained and the fluid sent for pathological testing. It must be emphasised that not all fluid around an implant is due to ALCL, but it can be a very stressful time for both patient and surgeon, until a diagnosis is made.

Not long before Christmas last year, Rachel called me, concerned that one breast seemed to be getting larger than the other. The following is her story told in her own words (with only minor editing).

Three-and-a-half years after having implants, I started to feel unwell and was not sure what was wrong. My right breast had, all of a sudden, filled up with fluid and I called Dr Linsell on his mobile. He asked me to come into his rooms to see him.

The consultation

Jacqui, Dr Linsell's executive assistant, fitted me in for an appointment and when I took my top off to show him my breasts, it was extremely clear that my right breast was at least double the size of my left. Dr Linsell explained this was most unusual and that we needed to rule out the possibility of ALCL which is a rare type of lymphoma with an association with textured breast implants. Dr Linsell wanted me to have a Fine Needle Aspiration (FNA) to remove the fluid and wanted it done before I could travel home. Dr Linsell explained to me what it involved and I broke down in tears because I was terrified. Jacqui walked with me to the radiologist and made sure

I was okay. Throughout the whole process, I had the support from both Dr Linsell and Jacqui and I can't thank them enough.

I had to wait one week for the fluid results to come back so that I would know whether I had ALCL or not. This was a difficult time. As soon as I got home, I did what most people would do – googled ALCL and then thought the worst, particularly when a few days later, my right breast filled up again.

After what felt like the longest week of my life, my results came back. They were clear of ALCL. That was a relief but even after it was drained a second time, it kept filling up. I ended up having my breast drained four times over a period of one month. Furthermore, I was on antibiotics which seemed to make me feel even more ill.

Reaching a difficult decision

I have a very active lifestyle and went from training at the gym five times a week to none at all. This took a huge toll on me mentally and physically, and we still didn't even know why it was happening. Dr Linsell thought it may be related to lifting weights in the gym and suggested that, if it didn't settle on its own, he may have to remove my implants.

Immediately, I thought of how I had felt for the last three-and-a-half years and said, 'There is no way. I can't have my implants removed.' My implants had given me my confidence back and I didn't want to lose that again. I had been the fittest and healthiest I had ever been in my life, enabling me to compete in three fitness bodybuilding competitions in the previous year. I felt removing my implants was not an option and I would do anything to try and fix the problem.

Dr Linsell put me in a sling for a fortnight. It helped with the fluid; however, as soon as I took it off and went back to the gym, the fluid returned. A few months passed and the more I used my right arm the more the fluid increased. What an emotional rollercoaster!

I then started to come to the understanding that I may need to have my implants removed. I hadn't felt myself this whole time, and not being able to go the gym, I began to gain weight. My health was deteriorating, which was affecting those around me. It got to the point where my husband said, 'I just want my old wife back again.' I agreed with him, then cried as I knew what had to happen. I made the heart-wrenching decision to have my implants removed.

Off I went to see Dr Linsell again to discuss my options. We agreed that my health was more important than having larger breasts and that removing the implants should restore my health so that I could be back to normal. After seven months of being ill, on and off antibiotics, and gaining a lot of weight, I knew I made the right choice. I do not regret ever having implants in the first place as they allowed me to feel confident and appreciate the importance of being healthy.

Once we had made the decision, my concern was that I would go back to having saggy breasts again, but Dr Linsell said it was possible to have a breast lift at the same time as removing the implants. I felt so relieved and grateful that I could have the lift. The next thing I knew, I was booked in and counting down the days till surgery again.

Day of surgery

The day of surgery arrived. I remember sitting in the car out the front of the hospital, with no makeup on, thinking, *Here we go again*. When Dr Linsell was measuring and drawing all over my breasts, I was not uncomfortable standing there in front of him and my husband. I had bared it all so many times by now, it wouldn't have bothered me if anyone had walked in. I realised that throughout the whole process, I still had my confidence and didn't care what others thought of me. I was so proud of myself for that.

Once again, as I lay in the middle of the operating theatre room, lights shining so brightly on me, Dr Linsell rushed over as I was about to be put to sleep. He held my hand as I drifted off under anaesthetic to ensure that I knew I was in safe hands again.

The second operation (*written by Malcolm*)

I accessed Rachel's implants through the original scars on her breasts and found a double capsule around each implant. The body normally forms a single layer of scar tissue (breast capsule) around an implant. If two capsules form, the implants keep slipping in the cavity, causing fluid to form. The implants were removed and a mastopexy (breast lift) was performed. Theatre time was two hours.

Post-op (*written by Rachel*)

The procedure was a day-case and I returned to Dr Linsell's rooms the following morning. He explained what he had done and then said, 'Let's take a look at your new breasts'. I wasn't sure what my new breasts would look like and the thought of looking at them in the mirror for the first time was overwhelming. I felt I had to mentally prepare myself for what I was about to see. It was a real mixture of emotions. I was feeling scared but also relieved and happy it was finally over.

When he removed the bra and padding, my chest felt so much lighter and I was happy to see two breasts the same size again; my new perky, smaller breasts. I clearly remember Dr Linsell saying, 'They are all you now.' It was such an emotional time.

Summing up

I am now six weeks post-surgery and can't wait to finally go back to the gym, back to my healthy lifestyle and begin to feel normal again.

Four years and two surgeries later, I have no regrets with either surgery. I love my smaller, perkier breasts.

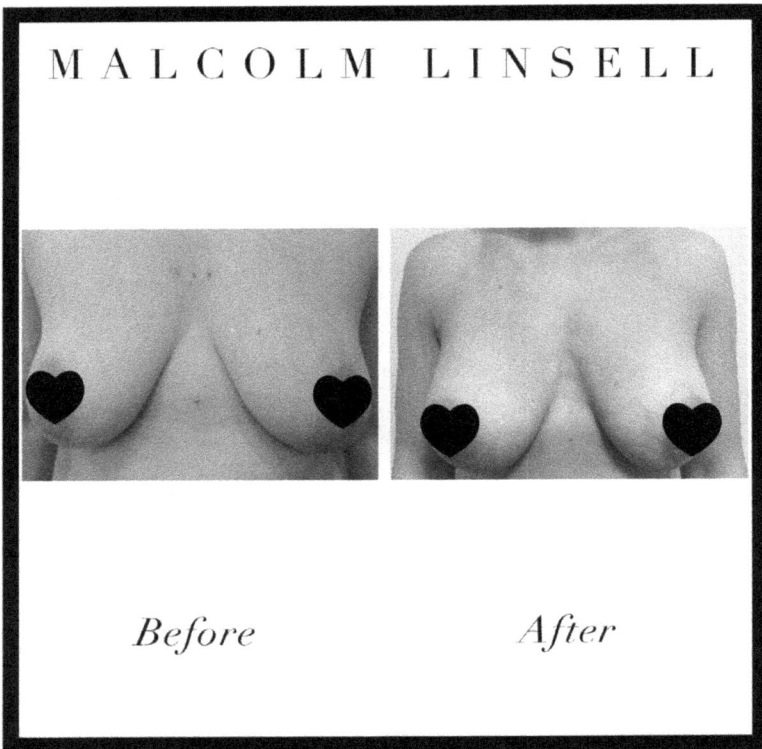

RACHEL: Before and after BREAST AUGMENTATION

MALCOLM LINSELL

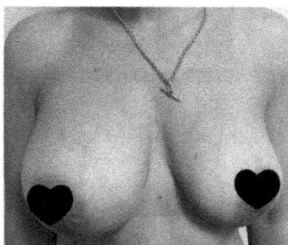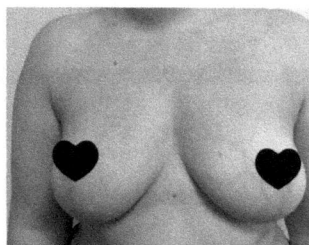

Before   *After*

RACHEL: *Enlarged right breast and after REMOVAL OF IMPLANTS AND LIFT*

LISA – Rhinoplasty, Tummy Tuck, Facelift, Blepharoplasty and Breast Reduction

Early life

Lisa is a twin, born in London UK, to working class parents. Although there wasn't a lot of money, there was always plenty of love and fun, with a great sense of family. Her childhood was happy, growing up in The New Forest, Hampshire, UK which still remains a habitat for many rare birds and animals. She was a little overweight and, as she took after her dad, she inherited his large nose. Compared with her twin sister, she felt she was the 'ugly twin' and her sister, Lauren, ensured she was frequently reminded of this. She completed her secondary schooling in the UK and took her General Certificate of Education O Level exams. She became a receptionist, then at the age of 19, immigrated to Australia with her first husband.

She has been a beauty consultant and now an account manager for a global beauty and fragrance company with 20 staff reporting to her.

Marriage and children

Lisa feels she and her first husband were never really on the same page and, after ten years, they separated. She remarried

24 years ago and she finds this marriage completely different. They are best friends, laugh a lot and have a total love and respect for each other, supporting each other with their joint and individual goals.

With her first husband, Lisa had two beautiful children, a girl and a boy, who are now aged in their 30s. She also now has three stepchildren.

Effects on her body and self

As a teenager and young woman, Lisa hated her nose, then after having her children, she didn't like her tummy with fat pockets that felt stuck to her hips. Later, around menopause, she didn't like her breasts which had become larger and saggy, and she felt that her face was looking tired.

As a young woman, Lisa hated how she looked, which made her miserable. She felt less confident in herself and worried about how others might judge her. She wore clothes trying to hide the parts of her body she didn't like, so the effect was less than flattering.

Considering cosmetic surgery

Lisa had wanted her nose fixed for many years. Her first husband was never a fan of 'changing yourself' but, at the age of 26, she got divorced and as a single woman, with some of her own money, no longer needed anybody else's permission.

She was living with her father at the time and talked about it with him. He told her to go and do it! She mentioned it to the man who was to become her second husband (although she didn't know it at the time) and he also was 100 per cent positive and supportive.

Lisa had a girlfriend who had just had a 'nose-job'. She liked what she saw, so made an appointment to see her surgeon to discuss the procedure of rhinoplasty.

The consultation

Before, during and after the consultation, Lisa was excited and relieved to be able to do something about how she looked. Her ideal outcome was for a shorter nose with no bump and the surgeon felt this was entirely achievable.

Following the consultation, she felt an overwhelming sense of relief and calmness.

Pre-surgery

Lisa feels the decision to proceed with cosmetic surgery on her nose had been made many years before she first saw the surgeon. As the time for her surgery drew near, she felt more excited because it would be the realisation of a dream for a more attractive nose. The only people she told she was moving forward with the procedure were the two men in her life. She didn't feel the need to justify her decision to anybody else. What she chose to do with her body was her own business and nobody else's. She knew the surgery would change how she felt about herself – in a good way – and that was all that mattered.

First and subsequent operations

Lisa's first operative procedure was a Rhinoplasty (nose job). Then, over a period of fifteen years, I performed several cosmetic enhancement surgeries, including a tummy tuck, followed by a facelift and upper blepharoplasty and, lastly, a breast reduction.

Then and now

Lisa is transformed. She is not the same woman, as she feels confident and proud of how she looks. This translates into the clothes she now wears, such as skinny jeans and more 'trendy' items.

Others notice. In fact, after her facelift, one of her work colleagues asked if she was having an affair as she looked so good and happy! Her husband thinks she looks fabulous, as do her children who are proud of how she presents herself.

She loves the fact that when she is naked, her body looks good – firm and everything where it should be.

A few months ago, I received a text from her which said she and her husband had just spent a week in Port Douglas. She said, 'I haven't worn a bra the whole time thanks to your brilliant work! I feel amazing and I am so grateful … xx'.

Summing up (*written by Lisa*)

'I look great, I feel great and I just love myself so much more! I am more confident in my personal and professional life. I am a better person for my husband, children, grandchildren, friends and work colleagues. This is all due to taking the steps I needed to follow, to change the things about myself (physically) I didn't like. I am emotional writing these words as the changes cosmetic surgery have given me are 100 per cent worth every cent I have paid – these procedures have repaid me ten-fold!'

One word to describe her experience … '*magnificent*'.

MALCOLM LINSELL

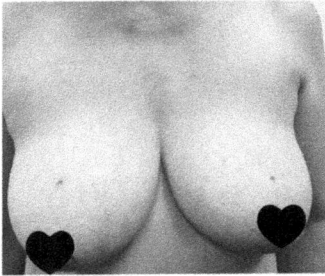 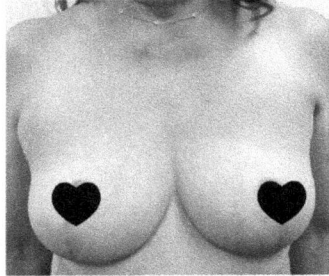

Before   *After*

LISA: Before and after BREAST REDUCTION

68

BIANCA – Tummy Tuck and Breast Reduction

Bianca's story is a little different because she has chosen not to have children. However, I believe her story will resonate with many, which is why it is included in this book.

Early life

Bianca was born and raised in Central Queensland. Along with her two sisters, she describes her childhood as the best because she grew up on the land. Her mum and dad and the three girls had an alternative, off-the-grid lifestyle, growing their own food.

Her mother was keen for the girls to have a good education. Having read books from an early age, Bianca enjoyed school and did well.

She worked at McDonalds, became a manager, then later changed track to be a real estate agent. She is now a beauty therapist, managing a beauty therapy business while also being a coach at a fitness centre, aiming to change the lives of all her clients. She loves both her jobs.

Marriage

Bianca has been with her partner for 13 years and, for the last four years, has been happily married. Their careers are important to both of them which requires them to spend a lot of time apart. This means they enjoy the limited time they have together. In this way they acknowledge and respect their mutual independence while knowing they are both loved.

One of the decisions they have made is to not have children. It is a life choice with which Bianca is very comfortable.

Considering cosmetic surgery

While in his mid-50s, Bianca's father died from cancer. This triggered her to change her lifestyle, lose weight and get fit. She worked hard to lose over 30 kg but found it difficult to reward herself. She couldn't wear a bikini or tight dresses as her belly would overhang, while her breasts were so large they seemed to take up her entire torso.

Bianca is a very confident person, but she couldn't get over the sadness her large drooping belly and hanging breasts gave her. She wore loose clothes to hide her body issues but no matter how much weight she lost, she still felt big.

She'd toyed with the idea of cosmetic surgery for about a year before booking the consultation. She researched tummy tucks online, but this made her hesitant because she knew she would be required to refrain from exercise while she was healing from the surgery.

One day, she had had enough. She discussed it with her husband and close girlfriends, who were overwhelmingly positive and excited that she could choose to do something that would make her happy.

After a recommendation from a friend, she made an appointment with our clinic. At that point, she stopped researching because she wanted factual information rather than being misled. She felt excited and a little bit nervous.

The consultation

Bianca was clear her ideal outcome was to feel good in her own skin, to know that her hard work had paid off and that she looked good. She was at ease, felt calm, knew that she had been listened to and understood, and felt that she was being cared for.

At the end of the consultation, Bianca was keen to book her procedure. The cost surprised her because she thought it would have been more expensive!

Pre-surgery

As the operation drew near, Bianca was excited. She just wanted to be on the other side. She felt proud to be doing something for herself, which she knew would make her feel better. Consequently, she did not keep her intention secret and was happy to share this with anyone who cared to ask.

Day of surgery

On the day of surgery, Bianca was relaxed. She had listened to me, read all the material she had been given, knew the risks and was comfortable with the decision she had made. She just wanted to wake up with her excess skin gone.

She was still relaxed as I was marking her up prior to the procedure, though she found the hospital cold. As always, I asked her what music she would like playing as she went off to sleep. She thought this was 'cute' but made her feel even more comfortable.

The operation

Bianca had a breast reduction followed by a tummy tuck with liposuction to the abdomen and hips. Theatre time was four hours.

Post-op

When Bianca woke, the first thing she remembered was that she was hungry. She had some pain which was easily controlled by the nursing staff in the recovery room. She rested for a while, had something to eat, then after I had seen her to make sure all was well, she went home.

Her first night was uneventful as she took her medication as directed, ate some dinner then went to sleep.

The first week

When Bianca saw her bruises and swelling on the first morning, she initially felt a bit light-headed, but felt better after her shower. She has a high pain threshold, so she felt that if she moved a little then rested, her pain would be kept to a minimum. She did little laps of the house, while keeping her body stretched upright.

Her husband was on hand to help, making sure she had food and took her medication on time. However, as previously mentioned, Bianca is quite independent, not wanting to rely on others too much. She sent her husband back to work on day three!

She knew the surgery had been worth it from day one. Any painful or negative thoughts were let go of immediately. She recited her affirmations daily and focused on the timeline she had set for her body to achieve specific things.

The next few weeks

Bianca was back to the gym as soon as the six-week mark ticked around. By three months, she felt back to normal but, as her exercise intensity increased, she had days which left her a bit swollen, so she had to modify her workouts.

Then and now

Bianca has always had a positive outlook but there were times in the past when her appearance upset her. Now, she is more in love with herself and how she looks. The baggy clothes designed to hide her imperfections have now changed to high-waisted numbers, bikinis, tight dresses and shirts, with midriff baring tops worn to the gym. Others have noticed how good she looks and how she presents herself.

Her husband loves her body and loves the confidence she has. When naked, she knows she looks good and finds that she enjoys looking at her body more.

Advice to other women

Bianca has no hesitation in recommending cosmetic surgery for others if they are considering it. She believes people will always have an opinion on what you do, but that is just *their* opinion. Focusing on what others say or do is of no benefit. However, if you are considering cosmetic surgery because you believe it will make you happier, enjoy your life or love yourself a little more, then go for it. The pain is not that bad and, if you take heed of the recovery process, you will be better than ever.

Summing up

Prior to the surgery, Bianca was worried she would struggle with not being able to exercise the way she was used to. For the short time she was out of action, she ate a very clean and healthy diet, so that when she got back into action, she had improved overall. She is very happy with her result and feels it has been totally worth it.

One word to describe her whole experience … 'amazing'.

M A L C O L M   L I N S E L L

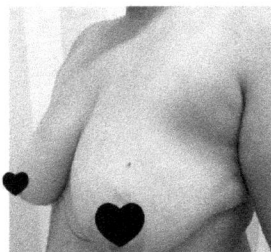

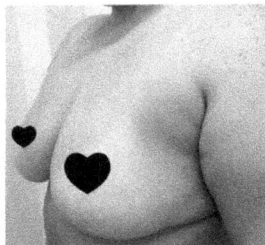

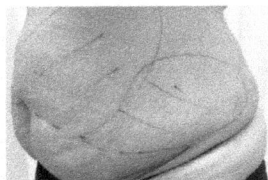

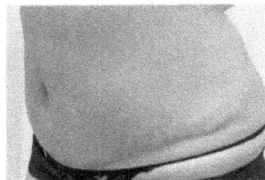

Before   *After*

BIANCA: *Before and after BREAST REDUCTION and TUMMY TUCK*

ERICA – Tummy Tuck and Fat Transfer to the Breasts

Erica has written her own story and it is reproduced below, with only minor editing.

My background

As a country girl, growing up in rural Victoria, my playing field was a dairy farm complete with push bikes, motor bikes and horses. My childhood was fun. I loved the open space of the country, the endless shenanigans with my cousins, the weekly footy and netball meets, and the freedom of just being a kid.

I'm the third daughter of four and our parents worked hard to support us all. They milked cows for a living and Dad also held down a job in town. Lavish items and extravagant holidays were few and far between, but I wouldn't change it for the world, for I feel that these years were invaluable for the person I would become.

When I was ten, our family packed up our belongings and relocated to Queensland for what I now know as home. I attended school in Central Queensland for both my primary and secondary years. I was never a model student. I never really applied myself as I cruised through life waiting for life to happen instead of making life happen.

After I finished school, I was initially a receptionist but when the opportunity to work with children arose, I threw myself at it headfirst. I felt this was my calling and still do. I'm not far off completing my degree in Bachelor of Education in Early Childhood, something that seemed so farfetched for a girl who, for so long, lacked clarity, motivation and determination.

I have a huge passion for helping others, in whatever capacity I can. For now, as a kindergarten teacher, knowing that I am helping to guide the lives of children during their most formative stage in life is extremely satisfying.

My family

I currently live in Central Queensland with my husband of 11 years and our three gorgeous children, aged six, seven and nine. I'm so lucky to be their mummy and each day I am amazed at how incredible they really are.

My siblings and parents live in Victoria. I miss them dearly, but I love the sun, and they are only a plane flight away.

My post-pregnancy body

Approximately ten years ago, when those magical two lines appeared on my pregnancy test, I was excited but really had no idea what to expect. Then, the changes started to happen to my body – the weight gain, the stretch marks, the love handles – you name it, I got them. Not only was I underprepared, I was faced with my greatest fears and there was nothing I could do about it.

Surely this was supposed to be the happiest time of my life, right?! Expecting my first baby, head over heels in love and planning my future. At times, it was. But then came the postnatal body and that was disappointing to say the least. I was now a mum, but never had I imagined myself looking or feeling the way I did. I felt defeated, consumed by darkness and embarrassed to be seen by anyone, including my husband. I tried to pretend that I was okay, that it didn't bother me, that everyone was like this in the beginning. I was wrong.

My mind never really accepted this look or feeling. With each pregnancy, my body image and mental state slipped further away from the person I wanted to be – the mother, friend, wife of those nearest and dearest to me. By my third and final delivery, anxiety, fear and depression seemed to consume me. It left me feeling worthless day after day, year after year. Every aspect of my life was centred around my physical image and the thought of being naked made me feel physically ill. I would never wear tight-fitting clothing, I would limit my food intake, I would exercise excessively, and yet it didn't change a thing.

My behaviour and relationships with others were greatly impacted as, in my head, I felt like I was not good enough.

Research and choosing a surgeon

My extensive research started after the arrival of our first daughter. Even though I knew I wanted more babies, I felt like I needed to be armed and ready to take action when the time was right. I spent countless hours researching plastic surgeons, looking at their credentials, photo galleries and, most importantly, internet reviews, because the honesty of previous patients can be very educational and persuasive.

The research gave me many highs and many lows. Sometimes, it would play with my mind and leave me asking questions such as, 'Am I vain?' or 'Why would I even consider this?' On paper, someone can look like the most amazing person in the universe but, in reality, they could be a jerk. Early in my research period, I met another local surgeon, booked in for an abdominoplasty, and tried to convince myself that he would give me the best outcome. While I knew deep down that everything about this surgeon was not right, I was so desperate to change the body I had, I was willing to sacrifice my safety. Thankfully, my husband gave me the truth I needed but didn't necessarily want to hear. I cancelled. I felt defeated and it took another five years to build up the courage to see another surgeon about a Mummy Makeover.

My 'take two' on surgeons was one of the hardest things I've ever done, as it mentally challenged everything about myself. This time, however, I not only had Dr Google on board readily providing positive feedback, I viewed an entire *60 Minutes* show featuring the surgeon himself, Dr Malcolm Linsell. The empathy, care and genuine compassion he showed during that entire show had me moved from the get-go. A box of tissues sat solidly on my lap as tear after tear streamed down my face.

I was mesmerised by the power and skills of one man, by his love and gratitude towards his patients, and how he optimised the best possible outcome for them. To be honest, I actually stalked his social media pages to check that Malcolm Linsell, the 'surgeon' off *60 Minutes*, was in fact the same surgeon who operated in my hometown. How could someone so talented offer his expertise and knowledge and be located just a few minutes away? For reasons which are clearer to me now, I am certainly privileged to have him here and hope he stays around for a while.

So that was it. I rang the number I got from the website, made the appointment and waited an agonising five weeks to meet someone who I believed to be a 'real-life hero'.

The day I met my surgeon

I paced up and down the carpark before heading through the doors of Queensland Plastic Surgery, double checking over my shoulder that no one saw me. I approached the desk, said my name and sat down in the waiting room. My heart rate was sky high, my palms were sweaty, and I had forgotten the reason I was there. As I sat there, legs crossed and swinging back and forth, I questioned myself and my intentions again. Then, the door opened, a man smiled at me and invited me through the door.

I sat down to the right of him, my bottom on the edge of the chair ready to make a run for it. He spoke to me. (I'm not even sure what he said as I was too busy trying to calm down the nerves.) He introduced himself as Malcolm and asked me what had brought me to see him today. He was kind and gentle, and I felt mesmerised by his empathy. I blurted out, 'Mummy Makeover,' in record speed, as he made notes on a piece of paper. He asked me what I disliked about my body and what I was looking to achieve.

Wow, now this was a question that nearly brought me to tears. How could I possibly explain to a stranger, all the things I hated about myself? It was impossible; the list was far too long. I was scared and grasped hold of the chair as I spoke. I began to tell Malcom that while I loved my children, I felt like I did not love my body. It was hard to articulate all the things that brought about great anxiety and not tear up at the same time. Malcolm listened, he wrote down everything I said, and he asked questions about me. I felt safe in his presence; the hard part was over. Or was it? Not quite …

After I explained all my dislikes to Malcolm, I then had to show him. Boy, was that hard! My chest, glowing red from embarrassment, was now on display with one of the top plastic surgeons in Australia gazing at it in close proximity. I was ashamed, embarrassed, helpless and afraid of what this man would think. Much to my relief, Malcolm gave me his honest opinion about both my chest and my tummy, and he assured me I could get the result I was after. In record time, I got dressed and met him back in the chair to the right of him.

He explained the ins and outs of the surgery and I let him know my expectations. Not once did he push a surgery date, nor did he sugarcoat anything about the surgery. He was blunt, in a nice way, but very blunt. He assured me I would have to take time for myself, take time out of the family unit to heal. At that point, I knew this would improve the recovery period and only benefit my healing. I wanted to cry, to hug Malcolm, to tell him I loved him at that point, for in that appointment, not only had he given me hope, he had empowered me to take that leap of faith. My heart rate now a cool 200 and fighting back tears, I shook Dr Malcolm's hand and headed for the door.

Dr Malcolm Linsell, you are truly one of a kind. I will be #forevergrateful for your wisdom, your kindness, and your genuine care for me as a person. You have an exceptional power that enables you to heal people from the inside to the outside and that, my friend, is exactly what you have achieved for me.

Booking and costs of surgery

I tossed about potential surgery dates, emailing backwards and forwards, trying every which way to find an excuse not to book it. Why? I've no idea, to be honest. I mean, I really wanted it, like *really* wanted it, but the fear of uncertainty was like a lingering dead animal that deterred me from looking beyond this. Here I was, this small-town country girl at heart, toying with the idea of plastic surgery. It really tested my morals and upbringing for some time.

However, one night I just told myself that this doesn't have to change my morals, but it sure can change my future, so I paid the deposit and the rest is history. For the first time in ten years I felt freedom. A sense of calmness had taken over my body and I was at ease with myself. What I do regret is that I booked the surgery without telling my husband. It was wrong, but I was so afraid that he might try to talk me out of it that I felt like I had no other choice.

It's hard to put a price tag on something so life-changing. It's kind of like buying a new car – do you just go with what is the 'best price' and hope for the best, or do you consider the quality of the overall product? For me, this was a no-brainer. Quality meant everything. I wanted the best possible outcome by the best possible surgeon, and I knew that any comparison with 'discount' procedures wasn't even on the same page. The costs associated with the surgery were appropriate for the great quality I received, and I had no objection in paying them. 'Quality is never an accident. It is always the result of intelligent effort' – John Ruskin.

So, who did I tell?

My little sister was the first person I told. After I booked my surgery, I rang her to share my exciting news. Her response was, 'OMG sista, that's so amazing. Do what makes you happy.'

Boy, that was a relief to hear. Not only did she support me, she encouraged me to go ahead with my surgery. I also told my husband and, for the majority of the six months leading up to surgery, they were the only two people who knew.

However, I needed some support with the kids, so three months prior to surgery, I called my dad, explained my procedure, and asked for his help. That same day, he booked his flights from Victoria to Queensland, and I knew he was more than capable of sticking to the extremely tight and overwhelming schedule that the children's school and extracurricular activities required.

One week prior to surgery, I decided to tell my best friend. I hadn't told her to this point, not because I thought she would think I was stupid, but because I really wanted to keep it a secret to protect me, to prevent any harmless messages or conversations to convince me to change my mind. As I expected, she was very supportive and I knew that if anything happened to me, she was my wing gal. She would be the one who watched over my children and told them things about me that only a best friend from high school would know.

As the months trickled down to weeks and days, I texted my little sister so she could share in my enthusiasm and excitement for my impending surgery. That she did beautifully, and I cannot ever thank her enough. #forevergratefullittlesister

The day of my surgery

At 5:00 am my alarm went off and I was like a racehorse running in the Melbourne Cup. My bags were packed; I was dressed in record speed and ready to leave 15 minutes later. The kids were asleep, but I rounded up my husband and my dad (who was in town for a week) and I pretty much ran to the car. The anticipation almost killed me, knowing that for so long I had dreamt of this day and it was finally here.

I checked in to the hospital, casually walking down the staircase, knowing my name could be called at any time, all the while with my husband by my side. Eventually, my name was called. I kissed my husband goodbye and told him, 'I've got this from here'. I answered a million questions, repeated my credentials at least seven times, showered and slipped into the hospital attire that not even Cindy Crawford could pull off.

When the call came in that I was next, I contemplated running to theatre without the trail of paperwork the staff were flailing around to find. It was there where, yet again, I was met with the same smile that Dr Linsell had greeted me with some months ago and my mind was put at ease. I knew it was okay and that I would be okay.

Then the hard part came – mark up time. Yep, sure I'll just display the most vulnerable parts of myself at close proximity to a world-class surgeon without any form of embarrassment … no way! I was terrified and had there been a syringe in sight, I would have administered the anaesthetic to myself right at that moment. The surgery itself didn't scare me, but the fact that I was fully conscious and half naked? That shit was hard. Really hard.

It was go-time. I rolled through those theatre doors and was ready to get the show underway. Malcolm calmly held my hand, asking who my favourite musician was, and then played my favourite song. He spoke to me like a friend, talking about AFL teams. I won't hold it against him that he's a Saints supporter and I don't think I could persuade him to change to barrack for Collingwood, but it was nice of him to take my mind off the procedure. He never let go of my hand and I felt comfortable and relaxed. I knew I was in the best hands possible.

When I woke up, I was on cloud nine, I couldn't feel a thing. There was no pain and I just wanted to go back to sleep. My husband was there, holding my hand, asking how I was. Communication at this point almost required an interpreter, but he smiled and that was all I needed. I had no concept of time, but I was comfortable, relaxed and very sleepy, so I took the chance to sleep.

Malcolm came around at some point and I asked some questions. What language that was in I'm still unsure, but nevertheless he answered them. He said it all went well and his words of advice were, 'Take it easy'. The nurses woke me some time later and asked me to go for a walk, and I knew that if I ate something, walked, and used the bathroom, I was a free woman. So that's exactly what I did. The idea of staying the night was not even considered. At 4:45 pm, I grabbed those discharge papers and headed for the doors. I walked all the way to the car and, again with my husband by my side, we headed for home. The first night's sleep was incredible – post-anaesthetic sleep is just so amazing – plus I had 20 pillows wedged every which way to catch me, support me and soothe me.

The operation (*written by Malcolm*)

Erica had a tummy tuck and liposuction of her abdomen and thighs. This fat was then transferred to the upper part of her breast and cleavage area. Theatre time was three hours.

Post-op – the first few weeks (*written by Erica*)

Week one: I expected the most incredible, insane, unmanageable pain. I had built up in my mind that this Mummy Makeover was going to be so painful that the world might actually end. To be honest, I was a little disappointed because it was far from that. In fact, the more I gently moved about, while following the rules, the easier the recovery was. I followed the directions to a tee, religiously drinking Sustagen hospital formula three times a day to enable the fat transfer to my breasts to survive. In fact, I felt like I had checked into a nursing home and that I was on a liquid diet. Nevertheless, I drank it, exhausting almost every flavour, but I did it because I wanted my newly plump breasts to remain just that!

Week two: Never sneeze or cough! The tightness of the sutures will confirm that your muscles are in fact stronger than ever and that Malcolm likes to create a finish that is tighter than a guitar string. However, movement was a lot easier and the abdominal binder was still very much loved.

Week three: The swelling was just damn right annoying, especially by the end of the day and the beginning of self-doubt began to creep in as I got a glimpse of my newly shaped tummy and the 30 cm incision line. At this point, comparisons to other Mummy Makeovers I found on the internet began to dominate my thoughts and create even more self-doubt. I began to wonder if I had made the right decision; was my incision too high, would it heal, would I get an infection? What if I had just made the worst decision ever?

This week was mentally the hardest for me. Cabin fever was real, and it really frustrated me that I couldn't do simple tasks that even my five year old could do. At this point, I couldn't even consider the new me because the way my tummy was looking was damn right depressing. My breasts on the other hand – well they were black and blue but damn they looked good and, even from the get-go, they never hurt or worried me at all.

Week four: The abdominal binder 24/7 really became a pain in the backside – toileting, showering, finding clothing that doesn't show it, and trying to sit for more than ten minutes was a challenge. This was the beginning of our love/hate relationship; the binder and I still had another three weeks left of wear. The swelling was still an issue and taking comparison photos regularly didn't really help the process at all.

Week five: This week things were looking better. I began to fight the mental battle of self-doubt and reminded myself that this was a process and that results do not happen overnight. This was also the week I decided to tell my mum and my other two sisters about my surgery. I no longer cared what people thought of me and I knew no one could change my mind, so I sent my sisters a few messages with some pictures and explained my surgery. They were so supportive. In fact, they even told me I was a brave person and that undergoing such a procedure takes great courage. I was relieved.

However, I still had to tell my mum and really wanted to do this in person. So, I did. I showed her some pictures and she was extremely happy for me. Finally, I was able to share my recovery with the people who meant the most to me, and that was life-changing.

Where I'm at now

I'm currently sitting at just over 12 weeks post-op of my Mummy Makeover transformation. Life is good – really good.

I have an abundance of confidence and each day I feel like I am getting closer to the person I always wanted to be. I've been working hard on my fitness and training to complete my first triathlon in over 17 years! I'm loving the fact that I can wear whatever I want and feel comfortable in doing so. Not only has this boosted my physical appearance, I am mentally a much stronger and wiser person. I no longer walk past the mirror and shudder at the reflection I see. I don't get hung up on small imperfections because I feel perfectly imperfect.

Each day, I wake up and reflect upon the new me and I start to make plans about my future. What hopes and dreams I have and what actions I need to take to make them my reality. I'm so determined to succeed in every aspect of my life, and I'm so thankful for the new me – the happy me and the me who has no limitations.

My relationship with my husband is stronger and I feel I am able to communicate on a deeper level. For the first time, I was able to explain to him how this surgery changed my life, my thought process, and my physical and mental status. It allowed me to be completely vulnerable, honest, laying out the naked truth about everything. It was a hard conversation, but nothing in life is easy, and I knew he needed to know about the old me so he could see just how amazing the new me really was.

I had a friend recently tell me that I am such a good influence on her life and how she told all her friends about me. While blushing at the time, I never really knew that simple words of encouragement, support and positivity could impact another's life so dramatically. This newly found confidence that I have, not only directly affects me and my family, it also is helping to empower and support my friends who in turn pass it on to their friends.

So, all in all, this remarkable surgery has had such an impact on my life that other people, who I don't even know, are feeling the benefits. For me, this is breathtaking and defines the power of positivity in its simplest form.

People from all aspects of my life and my children's life have compliment my appearance and said how incredible I look. More recently I was told I looked like a super model and, while I'm confident my modelling days are over, I was flattered by the remark. It just confirmed that I had made the best decision ever.

Has it been worth it?

Yes, yes and yes. The outcome I expected and the results I got were on point. I wanted a flatter tummy and perkier breasts. I got just that and so much more! My tummy is flat, shaped to perfection, and my breasts are plump and sit where they used to sit!!! I am over the moon, happy at the overall experience and, to be honest, I wish I had walked this road sooner.

To anyone considering cosmetic surgery, take a chance, for you might just surprise yourself. I did. It has been one of the most fulfilling things I have done. Leading up to my surgery, I relied on this quote a lot: 'What if I fall? Oh, but my darling, what if you fly?' – Erin Hanson. For me, I knew that the outcome outweighed the chance of falling and in my mind the only option was to fly. Fly high, reach new heights and continue to soar. That is exactly what I did and continue to do.

Dr Malcolm Linsell, you have played a significant role in helping me 'move mountains'. I am the absolute best version of me and will continue to build on this person for the rest of my life. Your wisdom, your skills, your compassion, your kindness and your genuine care for me have given me back the ability to create the life I always dreamt of. My journey is far from over and I'm taking every opportunity to fulfil everything I've put off over the years. Today, tomorrow, next week, next year, they are all my days, days that will empower me to move mountains and I'm well on my way to achieving greatness. #forevergrateful

MALCOLM LINSELL

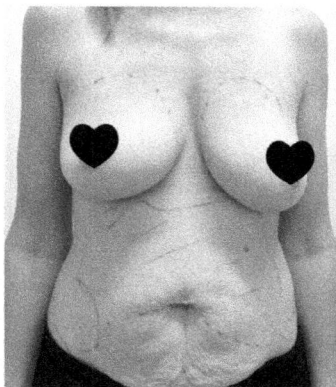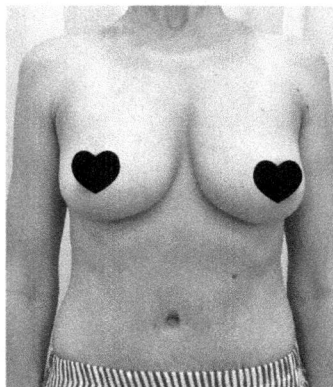

Before   *After*

ERICA: *Before and after TUMMY TUCK and*
FAT TRANSFER to the BREASTS

GENEVIEVE – Tummy Tuck, Breast Lift and Fat Transfer to the Breasts

Genevieve has written her own story and it is reproduced below, with only minor editing.

Early life

I was born in 1955 in Queensland. I was blessed with two sisters who I love dearly and, while I came in the middle, I cannot remember ever feeling the odd one out, or whatever the 'middle child syndrome' child should feel like.

Perhaps the greatest contribution to that was made by my mother, who has been the best mother ever. Having three girls under three, she invented ways that we would play together and have loads of fun, while she worked from home dressmaking for others. She would sit in a play pen with her sewing machine and we would play together outside that space. The 'play-names' she gave us were Josephine Mariah, Genevieve Anastasia and Lady Jayne Teresa.

My father worked hard as an auto mechanic and drove taxis at night, but was a Jack of all trades. He built our family home, which I have special memories of, in Toowoomba. Mum and Dad were of the Christian faith, attended church weekly, and were actively involved in many aspects of church life. When I was young and into my teenage years, the Christian faith was important to our family and it became very important to me personally. I believe the foundations of that upbringing gave me a solid awareness and belief in my value as a person, which has kept me in good stead throughout my life. I knew I was loved and that my life was significant, which built a confidence within the very core of my being.

I was a normal-sized child until the age of six or seven, when I started becoming 'chubby'. I remember Mum taking me to our local GP at the age of ten as my weight was increasing. My build was pear-shaped – heavy legs and bottom with a smaller waist and top. Having this shape did not encourage me to do a lot of sporting activities. So, from an early age, I was conscious of a weight phobia and I remember taking Vita-Weat biscuits and apples to school, while my skinny friends would eat the tuckshop food and snacks. It didn't seem fair, although, I was thankful that I had a 'pretty face' as people would say.

I've always been a 'girly girl', loving my hair well-styled and taking an interest in my grooming. I wanted to be a beautician from an early age. So at 15 years of age, I began an apprenticeship and, even before my graduation, I managed a hair and beauty business in the city of Brisbane.

It was at the salon that I met a woman who came to Australia to introduce Weight Watchers International. I joined up and learned how to eat 'proper food' with better combinations. I became a Weight Watchers Life Member. I was doing pretty well with my weight management though was not able to lose my 'tree trunk' legs and thick thighs.

I met a young man who I had known from childhood as our families had been acquainted in earlier years. Our romance began and we were married in 1977, celebrating our 43rd wedding anniversary this year.

The children

Our greatest gift has been our three children. They have all married now, and we love and cherish them, their partners and their children. At last count, we had four grandsons and two granddaughters.

We both have a strong Christian faith and are passionate about people and their spiritual wellbeing. This led my husband and me into Christian Ministry some 27 years ago and we have journeyed to many different cities, working together as a team with the same goals and heart. It has been a privilege and a good, compatible union.

Effects on her body

My husband has always shown love for me and I have felt treasured by him. He has witnessed my struggle with my weight fluctuations and my endless attempts to get fit. He's watched me trying to exercise to decrease the size of my legs ... joining gyms, walking, exercising and seeing dietitians. And he's seen the deep abiding disappointment of never having much at all to show for this effort.

My physical structure of knock knees and large legs, along with the osteoarthritis gene, has meant unreasonable stress on my knees. At age 51, I had my first knee replacement, followed by a spinal fusion, an ankle fusion and, last year, my other knee replaced. This has inhibited my physical activity in many ways.

Effects on herself

I have always chosen to look my best, despite my size, and over the years with fluctuating weight, I have worn many different styles of clothing. Of course, there are not many options in styles when restricted to the larger size fashions. But it has been important to me to present well and make the most of my good attributes. I had to come to terms with the fact that I would never be able to do much about my shape. Genetically, we are who we are. But my aim was to try to be as healthy as I could and to always present myself with every confidence in who I am as a person.

Considering cosmetic surgery

Malcolm has been a friend of ours since the 1980s when we moved to Melbourne. We journeyed with him through the years of his study and graduating as a plastic surgeon, and we have admired him as a friend, doctor and human being. His discipline and tenacity has always been incredible.

At the time of my first knee problems, my husband encouraged me to talk to Malcolm about potential cosmetic surgery. We wondered whether decreasing the size of the knee bulges and excess fatty tissue in the legs would help alleviate some of the stress on my knees and back. We also talked about a 'tummy tuck' as the three caesareans had left me a bit 'saggy baggy'. Back then these were the two areas of my body with which I was most dissatisfied.

At the time, the cost for these procedures was not affordable for us, so I put it away in my head as never going to happen. Fifteen years have passed since then – years of weight gain and weight loss, good fitness regimes and seasons of non-fitness. By 2015, I'd reached the heaviest weight I had ever been.

My husband and I faced many changes in our circumstances. Our fathers had both passed away within a seven-week period and it was a difficult and challenging time in our lives. I did not feel good about my weight and felt quietly depressed. By early 2016, I began at a new place of employment and commenced a better eating program and a more active life. My weight began to drop and my confidence built as I became more healthy. By 2018, I was reaching a weight that I had been 17 years earlier. I felt so proud of my efforts.

Something had happened though. With the 'weight gain– weight loss' roller coaster, my breasts and tummy were like sagging bags. I commented to my husband that if I had some money, I would consider going to see Malcolm again. I was then turning 63 and felt privately embarrassed by my shape.

We didn't talk further about it at the time but, before I knew it, my husband informed me that I had an appointment with Dr Linsell next week at 9 am.

The consultation

I went into a complete spin. I was so hesitant. I was only just recovering from a knee replacement. We were moving to another state in the new year to live and start new jobs. Yes, I could think of many excuses why the timing was not right, but I continued with the appointment plan.

My dad had left me a small inheritance and my husband wanted me to spend it on myself. 'Let's get your tent fixed up,' was how he put it. He felt my dad would be happy about that. And having watched me over decades working so hard for so little return, he felt I well and truly deserved it. He was so proud of me.

From the moment I talked on the phone to Malcom's receptionist, Jac, to walking into the practice in Richmond, I was made to feel as comfortable and relaxed as I could be. While still hesitant, my first visit with Malcolm gave me confidence – positive changes could be made for me.

Malcolm engaged with me to clarify my understanding of what the procedures would be and covered every piece of information I needed, along with checking any concerns and questions I might have. He suggested that I have an abdominoplasty to remove my tummy sag, some liposuction on areas of the legs, transferring fat to my breasts, while lifting them at the same time. I don't have big breasts and, even at this stage, I didn't feel I wanted to go bigger. I was happy to stay the same size but be a much better shape.

I was secretly excited while at the same time terrified at the thought, but in awe of the fact that this could even be achieved. Such mixed emotions.

Malcolm then sprung a suggestion on me. He had a date for the following week which freaked me out as I knew I had to make a decision swiftly and, looking back, I am glad. His quote arrived in an email that day which was to be the deciding factor for me. With much encouragement from my husband, including discussions about the logistics, I pressed PLAY to get the process underway.

Pre-surgery

It was then that, amidst the nervousness, the underlying excitement appeared. I felt guilty about this op, as we had never had much in the way of money, and I felt uncomfortable in some ways that I was spending this amount on myself.

Malcolm explained that this was a common emotion and that a lot of women feel this sense of guilt. He also explained that the other surgeries I'd had were necessary and that this one was different as I was choosing to do it. That made real sense to me. It helped me accept that it was alright to go ahead.

I decided to keep the procedure confidential. I felt it was very personal and, to this day, I have wanted to keep it that way. Other than a close friend who I stayed with for a week after the procedure, my sisters, and my husband and daughter, no one else knows.

I knew that, generally, people wouldn't notice as I had been losing weight for a long time. It is about how I feel about the way I look to myself and my husband that matters to me. I don't want a lot of attention and comments. I have never desired that. For me it is about myself and feeling terrific.

Day of surgery

The day of the operation was a whirl, which was good, as I did not have time to think about it a lot. Right up until I was on the operating table, it felt unreal that it was happening. The hospital was perfect for the procedure, small and intimate, with staff who supported and cared for me beautifully, always making me feel confident. Every person involved with my procedure seemed to go the extra mile and I found the overnight stay a breeze.

Because I had experienced many surgeries, I was not scared about the process once I hit the operating theatre. I felt so relieved when I was waking from the anaesthetic. It was done!!

The operation (*written by Malcolm*)

Genevieve firstly had a tummy tuck and liposuction of her abdomen and thighs. The fat was then transferred to her breasts to improve her cleavage and upper breast fullness, and a mastopexy lifted her breasts back to where they used to be. Theatre time was four hours.

Post-op (*written by Genevieve*)

There were no surprises with the post-op period, as the nursing staff were so supportive and caring, making sure that pain relief was administered appropriately. I was, however, surprised at how comfortable I did feel, even when I stood up. The overnight stay was helpful as it made me aware of how I was to function when leaving there for home.

I was able to go home with no drains, dissolving stitches, and simple instructions to shower and look after my wounds. I was to wear the provided garment, which fitted from under my breasts to my pelvic region, for a period of six weeks, keeping my abdomen firm and protected.

The first week

Because my husband was away interstate that week, I was able to stay with a good friend who looked after me. I could shower myself and do everything personally I needed to, but it was helpful to have someone support me with meals and be there if I needed someone. I am forever grateful to her.

I didn't find the procedures to my legs and breasts painful, but the abdominoplasty was a painful procedure. I was surprised at the length of the incision. I felt it was a little similar to my caesareans, where every move or cough or sneeze was very painful. It was hard to stand up straight, but I also knew that this pain would pass, and I believed it would all be worth it. I confess that I did wonder sometimes, *What was I thinking?*

It seems I was allergic to something, either one of the medications, or possibly the garment that I was wearing. I came out with an itchy rash which spread all over my torso. Malcolm suggested changing the antibiotic and I purchased a cream. I also found that wearing a cotton camisole under the garment seemed to protect my skin. There was good improvement and, to this day, I am not sure exactly what caused the reaction.

By the time a week came around, I was heading back to Richmond to visit Malcolm. He was very encouraging about how well everything had gone and how well it was all looking. I headed off, assured and encouraged to ring with any concerns or questions, and with a follow-up appointment in six weeks.

The next few weeks

As with any operation, each week became easier. I had taken two weeks away from work and returned in the third week with no problem.

For the six weeks that followed, I was required to wear the garment, only taking it off when I had my shower. Twice a week I used Bio-oil to massage the scars, then retaped the scars on the breasts and along the abdomen.

After six weeks, it was a milestone for me to be able to take the garment away. Relief! I was so pleased with my new look and continued for another four months to apply the oil and tape.

Before and now

It has been important to me over these six months since surgery to eat sensibly and make sure my weight is stable. I do not want to gain weight again and my discipline in this area I know needs to be strong. I know it will be a life-long goal for myself.

It is now six months since my surgery and my visits to Malcolm have been encouraging for us both. I refused to look at the before photos on my last visit. But the difference is trans-formational. I am so pleased with the result. I feel so much more confident and am enjoying wearing a different look in fashion. When I see myself in the mirror, I am still amazed at the difference before me.

For me, the weight loss has been a significant step to this new look. The cosmetic surgery is the 'icing on the cake' (which of course I do not want to eat!); the transformation in appearance, the artwork on the blank canvas.

I am so very pleased that I was encouraged to go ahead with this procedure and I cannot thank Malcolm enough for his good work and for his commitment to his patient care. And when I see documentaries on cosmetic surgery that have been a failure, I am ever thankful for his great gift and skill.

Summing up

Would I do it again? Yes, definitely. A word to describe the whole experience ... *'transformational'*.

If any new technical procedures come about to help with the leg area, let me know and I will be happy to be the model for you, Malcolm.

MALCOLM LINSELL

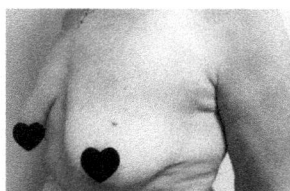 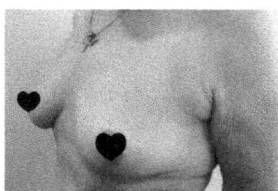

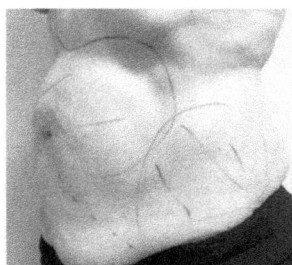 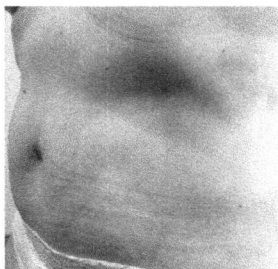

Before   *After*

GENEVIEVE: *Before and after TUMMY TUCK, BREAST LIFT and FAT TRANSFER to the BREASTS*

MONICA – Tummy Tuck, Breast Augmentation and Breast Lift

Early life

Monica's father was born in Italy, migrating to Sydney on his own at the age of 19. Her mother was born in Macedonia, escaping to nearby Austria during the war before migrating to Sydney with her family at age 10. Born in Sydney, Monica is the younger of two girls, her sister being 11 years older than her. When Monica was aged five, her parents divorced amicably, and she and her sister lived with their mother in a modest three-bedroom home.

When Monica's sister introduced her newly born twin boys to the home, space was at a premium. Monica's mother helped to raise the twins which occasionally led to strained relationships between the women. Consequently, Monica's childhood was not something she'd describe as particularly joyful and she learned to be independent from a young age.

While still at school, Monica found a job in retail as soon as she was legally allowed. She completed Year 12, then completed TAFE courses in Business Management and Graphic/Web Design. Between her twenties and thirties, she held several administrative and communication roles in the finance sector preparing her for her current role as a media officer.

The children

Monica has been married for five years and has two children, a son and a daughter under three. The family has moved interstate and has no family support close by.

Effects on her body

Monica's son was only ten months old when she became pregnant with her daughter, so there were three solid years of pregnancy and breastfeeding. This had a huge effect on her stomach and breasts. She had never been a slim girl, but she was fit. Once she finished breastfeeding, her breasts lost all volume. They became downward pointing triangles and she would often joke that she could tuck them into her socks. She ate healthily and exercised every day but, despite being back to her pre-baby weight, the bulge in her tummy hung down unless she clenched her abdominal muscles.

She enjoyed working out, but her stomach would wobble when she ran or jumped, causing her pants to fall down. She would constantly exercise without seeing any results, for no matter how hard she worked she always had an overhanging belly. Finding clothes to fit was a nightmare for her so she would wear flowy dresses or structured dresses that could hold her in. Pants were a no-go because of her 'swim ring' and the high-waisted skirts she used to wear remained in the closet collecting dust. She felt she could easily be mistaken for being six months pregnant.

She hated photos of herself and would delete them if her belly wasn't disguised. She hated having sex because she could see her breasts and belly hanging and jiggling which made her really self-conscious. Her self-esteem was negligible.

Considering cosmetic surgery

Monica had been dreaming about a tummy tuck ever since puberty had left her with noticeable stretch marks on her abdomen. Then, after her second (and final) child, she realised that no matter how much she changed her diet or slogged it out doing CrossFit or F45, the excess skin on her stomach and breasts, along with her separated stomach muscles, were there to stay.

She knew there had to be a solution so started researching risks and costs, looking at before and after photos and eventually found a Facebook support group for those thinking about surgery. Discovering so many women with the same body issues made her realise she wasn't alone. Watching them on their journey gave her the confidence and determination to start her own journey.

She shared her thoughts with her husband, who initially wasn't particularly receptive. He couldn't see the need and felt there were better uses for the money. Months went by and it was only when he realised how much Monica hated looking at herself that he switched to being fully supportive.

Monica continued to google, spoke with her GP, and contacted some of the local women on the Facebook support page. She had decided early on that travelling away from her children was not something she was willing to do. She lived in a regional city where there were only three surgeons performing the surgery locally. She felt that my reputation and experience far exceeded her expectations, so her choice of surgeon was made. Now, she felt excited and relieved knowing she was one step closer to her new body.

The consultation

The consultation was actually liberating for Monica because she learned that she was *normal*. She was reassured that her body issues were the result of growing and feeding two babies, not from lack of care or letting herself go.

She was able to clearly state that her desired outcome was for her excess skin to be removed, abdominal muscles put back together, a low abdominal incision line to be hidden by underwear, and natural-looking breasts in proportion to her body shape. She didn't want to stand out in any way; rather, she just wanted to look and feel 'normal' again.

I understood what she wanted and felt this was entirely achievable for her.

Pre-surgery

Monica was now excited she had made the right decision to have surgery. She had done her research, so the cost wasn't a surprise. She scheduled surgery between her work commitments and arranged for her mother to stay in order to look after the children, while she was recovering.

She kept the number of people who knew about the surgery to a few selected girlfriends. If more knew, she felt she may be judged harshly and didn't want to risk hearing any negativity.

Day of surgery

On the day, Monica felt a little nervous about being away from her children, but mostly she was just excited. This continued even as I was marking her up, for she knew that the bits that had bothered her for so long would shortly be corrected.

As she drifted off to sleep, she felt strangely calm.

The operation

Monica had silicone tear-drop shaped, textured implants placed beneath her chest muscle, to augment her breasts. This was followed by a tummy tuck with a small amount of liposuction of the tummy and hips. Theatre time was four hours.

Post-op

When she woke up in the recovery room, the first thing she became aware of was that she wasn't in any pain. That soon changed, particularly with the first time she got out of bed, but each time after that it got easier.

The first time she looked down, she knew it had been worth it.

Monica chose to stay overnight in hospital. She had birthed both of her babies at that hospital so, to her, it felt a little like home. With two toddlers at home and well cared for, she loved being able to recover in hospital knowing that, if anything went wrong, she was just a buzz away from help.

The first few weeks

After I had seen her the next morning, Monica went home. Her mother had come to stay for three weeks, particularly to look after the kids, and the first week was a lot easier than Monica had expected. By day five, she was walking around the local fruit and vegetable market with the kids. Her mother and husband were both astounded at how easy her recovery was. By week three, Monica could do everything by herself, so she enjoyed spending time with her mother, having lunches and shopping.

Then and now

Monica felt back to normal by six weeks. At the time of writing it is three months since her operation.

She feels her before and after photos are so different that it's hard to believe the 'before' was ever her. To her, everything just looked so … sad! She now loves her body so much more.

She has noticed that she has a stronger core and can hold positions in Pilates and yoga for longer. Her pelvic floor is stronger and although not back to pre-baby strength, it is far better than what it was. She has more shape and stands taller, with better posture.

Others have commented on how well she looks, but most have no idea she has had surgery.

Her husband has said how happy he is that she's happy with herself. He also seems to be a very big fan of her flat stomach and perky breasts. ☺

When she is naked, she notices that she stands taller and pushes her shoulders back more. Furthermore, she can lean over without seeing what appears to be a set of old socks hanging where her breasts should be. A bad choice of tattoo she had while in Thailand is no longer there because it was removed with the excess skin on her abdomen. She can now actually see muscle definition on her stomach and her pubic area no longer has a belly hanging over it. She likes what she sees now and is in no hurry to put her clothes back on.

Clothes

When asked about the clothes she can now wear, Monica said, 'One can never underestimate the pure joy in wearing a tight white top with a pair of skinny jeans, without overhang! I am also back wearing the high-waisted skirts I love, and I've even rocked a bikini a couple of times'. This makes her happy and confident. 'As a mum and a wife who is also trying to juggle her career, I don't have time anymore to hate myself.'

The changes in her body have given her the confidence she was lacking. She now feels she can get on with life. Between work, kids, the home and her husband, she feels her life is crazy. However, she feels it's just nice not to worry about how she looks or what she's going to wear to cover her belly. It's one less thing she has to worry about.

Furthermore, she no longer has the fear that people are going to say, *'Awwww, how far along are you?'* because, finally, she no longer looks pregnant.

Advice to other women

Monica's advice for other women considering cosmetic surgery is, 'Research as much as you can. Don't go with the cheapest option, go with the best surgeon. Be clear on what you want and ask as many questions as you need to feel 100 per cent comfortable and confident. Trust your surgeon who probably has several decades worth of studying and experience up their sleeve over anyone on a Facebook group'.

Summing up

Monica says, 'It's strange, because after having a baby I had so much admiration for my body. It's ability to create an entire human being, to create an organ in order to feed this human, and then dispose of it after the birth, then producing milk to feed the child (and create its own antibodies) is all such a mind-blowingly beautiful and amazing thing.

'Despite all of this, I still wanted my old body back. Now I feel like I have my old body again, but it's even more remarkable because it grew and fed my babies.'

Her one word to describe the whole experience ... '*fulfilling*'.

MALCOLM LINSELL

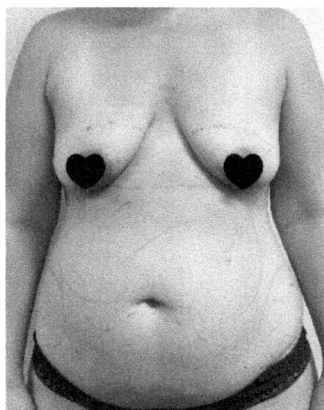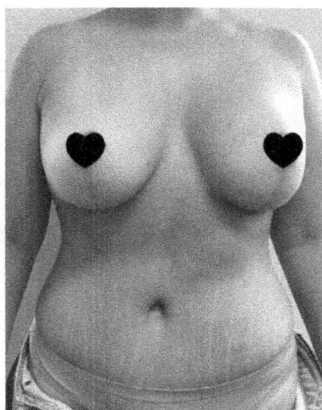

Before   After

MONICA: Before and after TUMMY TUCK, BREAST AUGMENTATION and LIFT

JENNY – Tummy Tuck and Breast Reduction

Early life

Born and raised in country Victoria, Jenny was the second eldest of four children. Many aspects of her childhood were unhappy. She was never close to her mother, who described her as her 'challenge' child. While her mother was not physically abusive, she was absent so that Jenny has no memories of doing anything with, or learning from, her mother. There were no bedtime stories, no playing Barbies, in fact, nothing that could be described as fun.

On the other hand, Jenny has very fond memories of the times spent with her father. On his days off work, or after work in summer, she would go running with her dad. They would run five kilometres each day together. Jenny was only seven years old when she ran her first 6.2 kilometre fun run with her dad. He taught her to use tools and mow the lawns, how to paint, how to make a flying fox on the 100-year-old oak tree where they lived. When she was nine or ten Jenny remembers riding on his motorbike with him. She always loved being outdoors with her dad.

Jenny and her older sister often conflicted with each other. Jenny was bullied frequently at the Christian school she attended and, while she does not recall her older sister joining in, she refrained from defending her. She loved to learn but hated school for it was never a place where she felt safe. She left the Christian school and attended a state school. The bullying became worse and, on top of this, she was sexually abused.

When she was 16, Jenny moved out of home and, while still at school, began work in a supermarket to support herself. Shortly after, her parents separated and Jenny moved interstate with a friend, completing her final two years of school by correspondence.

With the emotional neglect she experienced at home, combined with the bullying at school, Jenny developed a 'strong-willed' personality. She became a strong, independent child, young lady and woman discovering that she frequently had to 'fend for herself'.

She had always wanted to be a police officer and at the age of 15 did some work experience at a police station. She would have loved to join the police force there and then, but the timing wasn't right. She later worked in sales, then as a personal assistant, before being accepted into the police academy at age 26, a single mother of two children aged four and five. She is now a senior constable of the Victoria Police, working in general duties and first response.

Marriage and children

Jenny's first marriage was to a closet alcoholic. When he was sober, they had a lot of fun together. However, the drinking was excessive and, when drunk, he forced himself on her, which was almost every day. As they were both from Christian families, they had not lived together before they were married, so within three months of marrying him, Jenny was shocked and scared. She felt very much alone, abandoned, even by her own family. Although she was close to her dad, he was in a relationship himself with a typical 'wicked step-mum' type lady.

Jenny's marriage lasted three years and, in that time, she had two children. In hindsight and after many years of self-reflection, Jenny admits she married her first husband for the wrong reasons, thinking she needed a man to make her feel like she belonged to a family.

Two years later, she met the man who was to become her second husband. Their wedding day was the best day of her life (aside from having her first two children). It was a perfect day that went off without a hitch. She admits, they had their life 'issues', but 'who didn't'? Early on, Jenny saw no signs of abusive traits in her husband.

Three months after their wedding he was made redundant. Four weeks later, Jenny had a miscarriage, for which he blamed himself. Jenny grieved deeply over their much-wanted and planned-for baby (her third – his first).

Thereafter, he struggled with employment and she was unable to fall pregnant. After some tests, they learned his sperm was deformed. His self-worth had already taken a hit with the redundancy and miscarriage. This news had him spiralling further into depression. The worse he got, the more abusive he became to the family.

They had been told it was unlikely they could have another child without IVF treatment. It was therefore a surprise for Jenny to discover she was pregnant, just at the time she recognised there were some major issues with his treatment of her children and her. She justified and excused his behaviour until she was pregnant with her fourth (his second), and he was diagnosed with Asperger's. His behaviour failed to improve which significantly impacted her and all four of their children.

Jenny left the marriage when their youngest was five months old, processing her own grief, guilt and struggles with yet another failed marriage.

She now has four beautiful children, a 14-year-old girl, a 13-year-old boy, a 5-year-old autistic girl and a 4-year-old boy.

Effects on her body

Jenny hated her breasts and her stomach. She was an early developer with her first period at age 10. She was a D-cup breast from the age of 12, which was largely why she was targeted at school. Boys would constantly try to touch her breasts. She was ridiculed, bullied, ogled and sexually assaulted because of her breasts. Her love of running disappeared rapidly because 'they' would run alongside her or position themselves at the finish line where she could see them with their hands in their jumpers, mimicking her breasts 'bouncing' up and down. As a 14-year-old girl she recalls crying, with a knife held at her breasts, begging her mother to cut them off. Emotionally, it was an incredibly painful time for her.

At that early age, her mother took her to see a breast surgeon, but he refused to do any operation. He said she would 'grow into them'. Jenny was devastated. She became more depressed and hated herself. She developed an eating disorder, bulimia, in a fruitless attempt to gain control over her body.

Yet, the same breasts she hated, fed her four children for an extended period. Furthermore, as she had an oversupply of milk, she was able to donate milk to a premature baby, born three days after her third child. This saved that small child's life. Jenny was proud of what her breasts had done for those five precious children.

After her fourth and final child, Jenny lost 27 kg. However, her stomach became a massive problem for her. She felt she looked five months pregnant irrespective of how much weight she lost. She could not get rid of that tummy.

Consequently, she had never worn the clothes she wanted to wear. She is a runner with an athletic build, very stocky and incredibly strong. Yet she was always in baggy clothes, covering herself. Instead of feeling strong and toned, she felt overweight. For Jenny, it was a constant battle. In fact, clothes shopping had been traumatic from the age of 12. Every single time she 'had' to go bathers or bra shopping, she would end up in tears, sometimes sobbing on the change room floor. She hated every moment of it.

When she was 28 years old, she went bra shopping in Victoria's Secret in America. Jenny just wanted to feel sexy but warned the shop assistant of her previous traumatic experiences. She tried on about eight different bras until they found one that was a perfect fit. So perfect – she loved it and bought one in every colour! She came back to Australia with 12 different coloured bras in that same style.

Jenny struggled with conflicting emotions. She was proud of what her body had done in giving birth to four children yet despised it at the same time. She wanted this to change because she was raising two daughters and did not want them to struggle with similar self-image issues. Furthermore, she was raising her boys to love women no matter how they looked while, at the same time, respecting a woman's right to love herself in her own way. Her children never knew she hated her body but she was determined to prevent them from feeling the same way about themselves.

Considering cosmetic surgery

At 14, when Jenny had seen the surgeon about getting a breast reduction, her mother had gone through the motions of helping but didn't really understand how much Jenny was struggling as a large-breasted young woman.

After her first two children at the age of 24, Jenny saw a surgeon again regarding the procedure, but she was a single mum and couldn't afford the costs at that time. She knew she would have to wait a bit longer.

Nine years later, after another two children, and again as a single mother, Jenny decided the time was right. She was struggling with the sports she knew she could do but the size of her breasts and tummy were getting in the way. They were holding her back from achieving her physical goals and she knew she needed to increase her own self-love and worth. She worried others might think she was vain for having surgery, but knew she needed to do it for herself.

She spoke with her GP who was supportive and joined some Facebook groups for women interested in breast reduction. She valued the input and experiences of other women. She spoke with her older children who were 10 and 11 years old, explaining she needed help to relieve her migraines and back pain. They were also supportive and committed to looking after the younger children who at that stage were 18 months and 2 ½ years old. As she said, 'I was *done* with giving my body to babies and this was now my time to take care of me!'

The consultation

At the consultation, Jenny was initially nervous. She was excited because she had waited so long for this opportunity, yet her feelings were tempered with shame. As I spent time asking her about the outcome she wanted, Jenny started to relax because she began to realise that 'this could actually be happening'. Her dream could actually become her reality. By the end of the consultation, she felt elated.

Pre-surgery

Jenny didn't hide the fact she was proceeding with surgery. She was after a dramatic change, which she felt would be obvious post-operation, so saw no need to hide it. She told me that others don't hide the fact they have a new haircut, or a new job, or a new car, so she had no hesitation to inform those who needed to know.

As the day of surgery drew near, Jenny became more nervous, not because of any regret, but because of the risk of complications. Like so many mothers with young children, she was worried she would die on the operating table.

Day of surgery

On the day of surgery, Jenny wanted to cry. She was so excited and couldn't believe it was actually happening. As I was marking her up, she felt teary, knowing she was ready but she was scared at the same time.

However, once she was on the operating table, as she was being put off to sleep, I held her hand and asked her to describe her dream bikini and the dream holiday destination where she would wear it. This reinforced for her that this was her journey, her time, and as she drifted off to sleep, she knew this would be the best experience of her life.

Operative procedure

Jenny had a breast reduction immediately followed by a tummy tuck, which included some liposuction of her tummy and hips. At the same time her umbilical hernia was fixed. Theatre time was four hours.

Post-op

When she woke, her first feeling was relief. She was alive. She had no pain and couldn't wait to see her new appearance. Already, even with the dressings, she could tell how much smaller her breasts were.

As a single mum with four children at home, Jenny chose to stay in hospital for three nights to get the rest she needed for when she got home.

I took the dressings down the day after surgery. As soon as she saw herself and the difference in her tummy and breasts Jenny knew she wasn't going to regret it. She knew she was going to love herself in a different way – a way she had wanted to for as long as she could remember.

The first few weeks

Jenny was surprised with how well she coped at home. Her pain was not as bad as she had thought, but then again, she knows she has a high pain tolerance. Her older children helped look after the younger ones and although they were separated, her second husband stayed for a week to help. In retrospect, she feels this wasn't really necessary. She had prepared frozen meals prior to surgery. Her youngest, at 18 months old, was able to climb up onto the change table with her help or the help of the big kids.

In her recovery, it was fatigue that held her back the most, not being able to get through the day without a nap. As a woman who was always on the go and very active – and as a single mum – she found it challenging to feel so tired. Nevertheless, as a typical super-mum, Jenny just managed. She did it.

Five weeks and five days after her procedure, she ran her first five kilometres. She tells me it was slow! Then by nine weeks post-operation she felt back to normal.

Then and now

Two and a half years later, Jenny is doing things, wearing things and appreciating herself in ways she could only dream of before. She feels confident and strong, carries herself differently, speaks about herself differently and genuinely cares for herself. Interestingly, her ex-husband, who was initially supportive, became obsessed with her new shape and confidence. He became jealous that he was 'not sharing in her new body' and the result was a dramatic deterioration in their relationship.

Her children are a different story. They are proud of their mum. Jenny went on a holiday with her eldest children 11 months after her surgery. She was wearing her dream purple bikini, going on water slides with her son. She saw her daughter talking to a woman stranger and went up to see if she was okay. The woman told her, 'I cannot believe you have four children – your daughter told me you have four! Gosh, I wish I was as fit as you!' Jenny's daughter said that made her proud. She has secretly filmed videos of Jenny training and posted them on her Instagram, saying how proud she is of what her mum can physically do. Her son wrestles with her and loves it. While her younger two are too little to understand, her older two have seen the change in her physical capabilities and confidence.

Jenny considered getting a tattoo to cover the scar on her tummy, but her oldest son said, 'Mum, don't cover it. It's part of your journey'. She loved that he thought like that – and he is only 13!

When naked, she no longer hates what she sees. When she sees her scars, she smiles. As they fade, they remind her of how far she has come.

Clothes

Jenny now wears her bikini. She can wear backless dresses, thin straps or crop tops if she wants to. She wears fitted clothing as she's no longer trying to hide her body. Others notice. She is told that she is 'dressed up' a lot. She's not – she is just dressing the way she wants and that makes her feel good. She now has a different, increased, yet humble way of taking pride in her appearance.

Advice to other women

Jenny's advice for other women considering cosmetic surgery is, 'Don't wait. Find a way. If you want it – go get it! You are worthy of it and you are the only one who has to live IN your body. Do it for yourself and no one else!'

'I would also like to talk about the people I lost in my life because of this surgery. There are people – no matter what you do in your life – who cannot celebrate your happiness. That is their issue – not yours. I lost friends because they were jealous. I no longer speak to my mother because she told me I was a selfish mother for having the surgery, that I should've waited. I asked her, 'Waited for what? Until *you* were comfortable for me to be happy with my own body? This is not your journey'. Considering she took me to see a surgeon at age 14, her reaction surprised and hurt me more than any. But I have found that changing my body gave me the confidence to set boundaries, even with my mother. It was a turning point for me when I understood some relationships needed to be let go, that those people were never going to support me if I was happier than them. It is not my responsibility to carry that anymore.'

'My youngest son was 18 months old when I stopped breast-feeding him to have my surgery. My children went without nothing. This surgery did not make them miss out on anything else – but they gained a happy and confident mother who is so active with them now because she CAN BE.'

'You will likely lose relationships because of the surgery. People may judge you for many reasons – but always remember that their judgement is a reflection of their issues. Not yours.'

Summing up

Her one word to describe the whole experience ... *'life-changing'*.

Postlude

On a Sunday afternoon about 18 months after Jenny's surgery, I was relaxing at home. The last time I had seen Jenny was about six months previously, when she had told me she was retraining her brain to be confident with herself and enjoy the compliments she was receiving from others. Both she and I were delighted with her new size and shape.

I received a text from her, '... just wanted to share with you that I just finished my first ever marathon!!' She had just completed the Gold Coast Marathon and the text included a photograph of her triumphantly crossing the finishing line. This photograph is included on page 118 and Jenny is also featured on the front cover of this book.

What a magnificent and heroic achievement! Abused as a child, she gave up running because of the ridicule she had to endure, then gave birth to, and raised, four children as a single mother. Then, while still enduring criticism from significant people in her life, she had the *courage* to transform her body, creating for herself more *comfort* (no more back, neck and shoulder ache or bulging tummy), more *choice* (no more covering up with clothes, instead, wearing whatever she wants) and a boost in *confidence* that has dramatically transformed her life, but is also positively impacting her children and those around her.

MALCOLM LINSELL

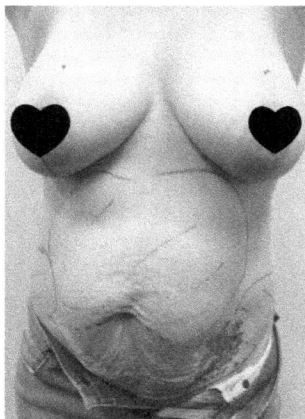
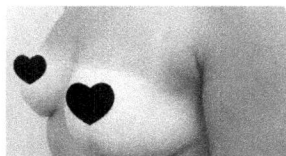
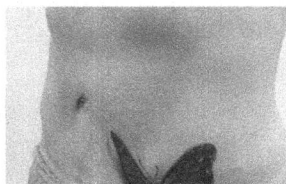

Before   *After*

JENNY: *Before and after TUMMY TUCK and BREAST REDUCTION*

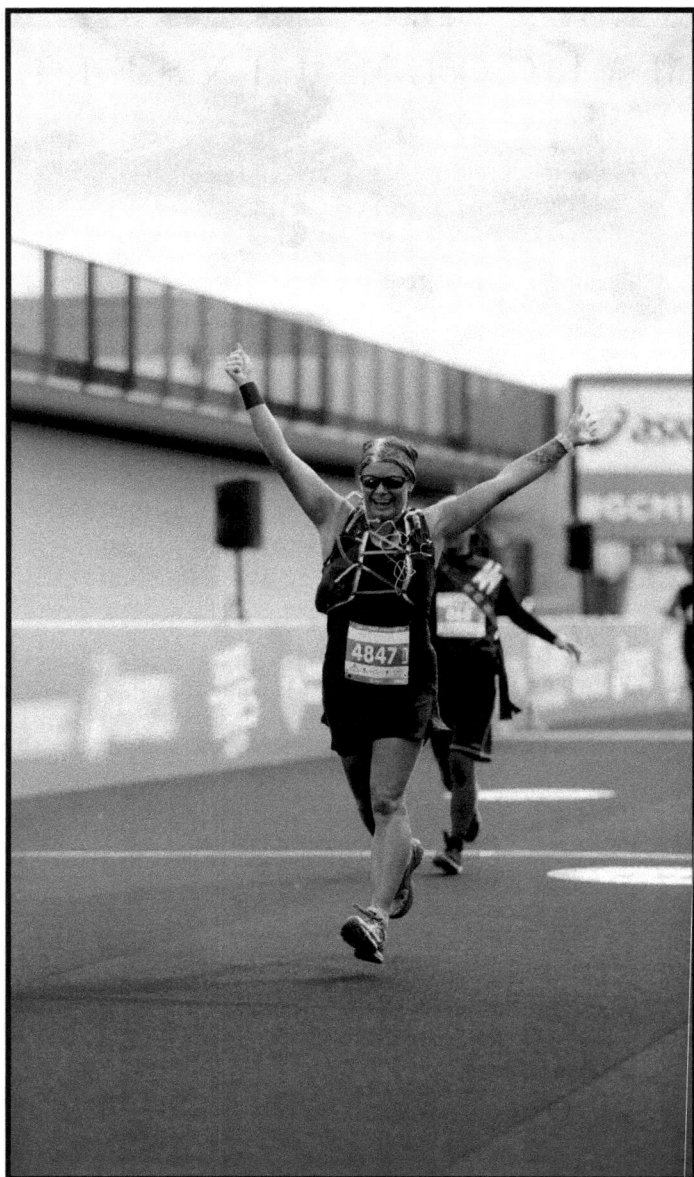

Conclusion

Every woman you have read about in this book is real. Their stories are as they told them to me and only their names have been changed. They have been open and honest and their stories raw. As you have read, they come from different walks of life, with different upbringings and life experiences. Yet they all (other than Bianca) share the common experience of having children and finding their post-pregnancy bodies had a negative impact on their self-esteem. Similarly, they share the experience of having the courage to undergo plastic surgery and find this transforms how they feel about themselves and their relationships with others. Yet, they have not stopped being real. All the before and after photographs displayed in this book have been taken by me and have not been digitally altered.

Over recent months there has been a groundswell in approval for social media posts to become more honest and real. I approve of Instagram blocking the use of augmented reality filters that depict or promote cosmetic surgery. This is a small step in what is a largely unregulated area of social media images.

Not everything you see on social media, and in fact in magazines, advertising, billboards etc., is real. For years, celebrities have used the very best makeup, hair styling, lighting and custom-fitting clothes, and their images have been taken by the very best photographers. Then their appearance can be digitally altered to remove any perceived irregularities to maintain their seemingly ageless appearance. Celebrities entertain and often inspire us, so is it any wonder that the use of a filtered image is now a universal accompaniment of a social media post? My concern is that we may become more attached to our filtered image of ourselves, rather than the real thing.

A friend of mine is an expert injector of facial fillers. Recently, she used filler to augment a young woman's lips and took a photograph of the result. She showed the before and after images to her patient who flatly denied the post-filler photograph, just taken, was actually her. 'That's not me!' she said. At which, she took the phone, held it elevated at the right angle, took her own image, adjusted it with a filter and then proudly exclaimed, 'This is me!'

There is some hope. I am writing during the pandemic caused by the COVID-19 virus. Much of the world is in lockdown and many are suffering. Some celebrities have made disastrous attempts to make us feel better by indicating, 'We are all in this together', when it is clear their privileged circumstances are diametrically opposed to most of the rest of the world. Yet, some celebrities have managed to connect with us just by being real. How this will play out in a post-COVID world is difficult to predict, but I wouldn't be surprised if there is some push-back from the public for celebrities to be more real with their images and posts.

At the beginning of this book, I said I love to make a difference in people's lives. When I hear a woman say that she can now wear the clothes she wants, that she doesn't have to think about what she wears, that she can go without a bra if she wants to, that she feels in proportion, that she can wear a bikini or one-piece swimming costume without feeling self-conscious, that she can wear a backless, strapless dress or a tee-shirt and jeans and feel comfortable, I know I have given her what she wants and that it has made a difference in her life. In fact, even without asking her, I can usually tell how she feels because I can see it in her smile.

Just yesterday, I was reviewing a lovely young mother of three children. She had undergone a breast augmentation two years previously and she loved her new breasts. I mentioned that I was about to publish my second book entitled, *I Love My Kids But I Want My Body Back*. She told me that is exactly how she had felt prior to her operation and I asked her to expand on what she meant. She struggled to put it into words but, as a younger woman, prior to pregnancy, she hadn't given a great deal of thought to her body. She had taken it for granted. Pregnancy, however, changed her body dramatically. In particular her breasts deflated and drooped and, while she loved her children deeply, she felt something had been taken away from her. She didn't feel feminine, she didn't feel sexy and her confidence diminished.

Nowadays, two years after her operation, those feelings are a distant memory. I asked her to compare herself now with how she felt as a younger woman, before pregnancy. Without hesitation, she replied, 'Better!' She went on to explain that now she was a confident woman who embraced her femininity with the added benefit of three children she had brought into the world and was helping to raise. It was like she felt complete, whole. Restoring her body was the final piece of the jigsaw. She feels complete and is loving life.

She and so many others have had the courage to transform their bodies and created for themselves more comfort, more choice and a boost in self-confidence that has made a difference in their lives and in the lives of those around them.

For me, to be involved in that process is one of the greatest gifts I can imagine.

Malcolm Linsell
Sydney, NSW Australia; Rockhampton, QLD Australia
September 2020

NOTE: If you are interested to know more, you are invited to follow me on Instagram @drmalcolmlinsell or visit my website at www.drmalcolmlinsell.com.

I can be contacted by email on malcolm@drmalcolmlinsell.com.

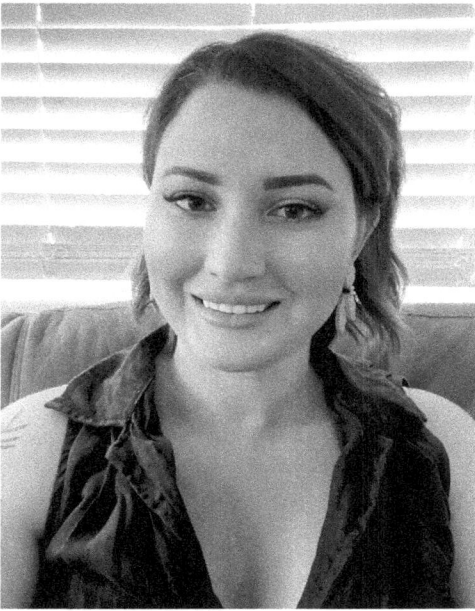

Chelsea

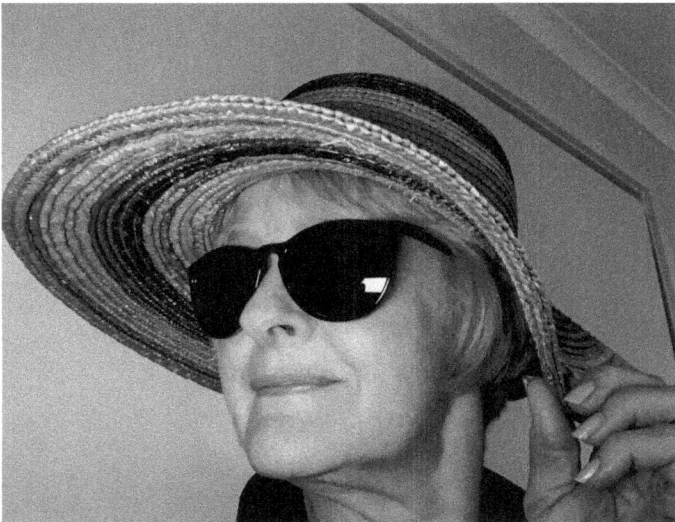

Genevieve

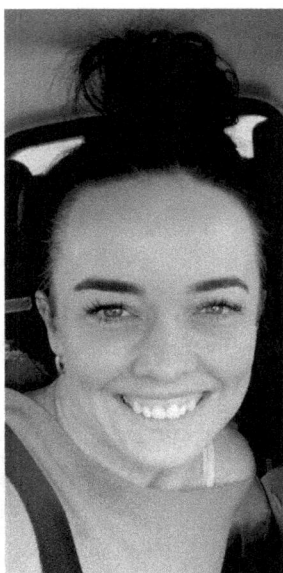

Rachel

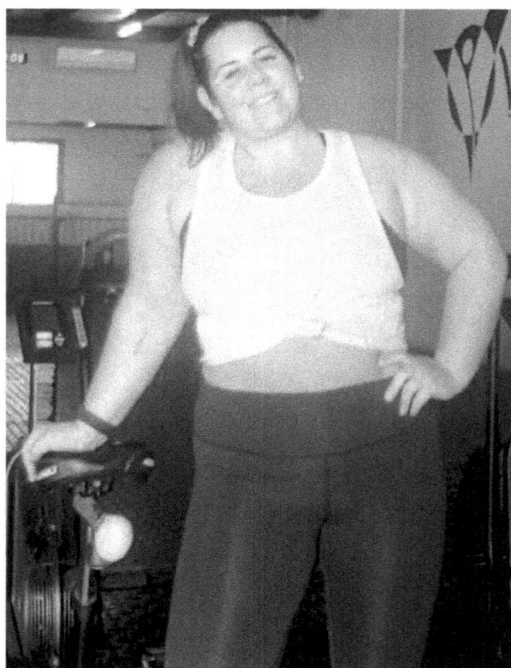

Bianca

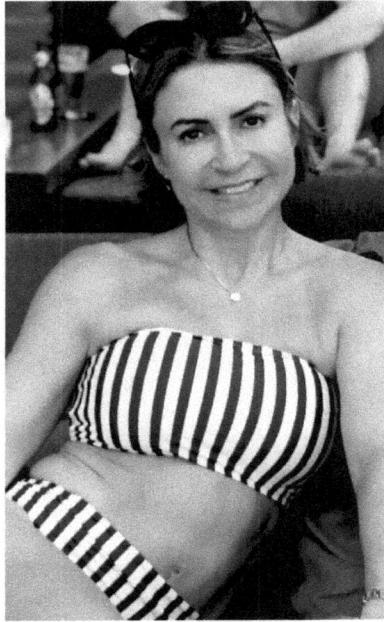

Julia

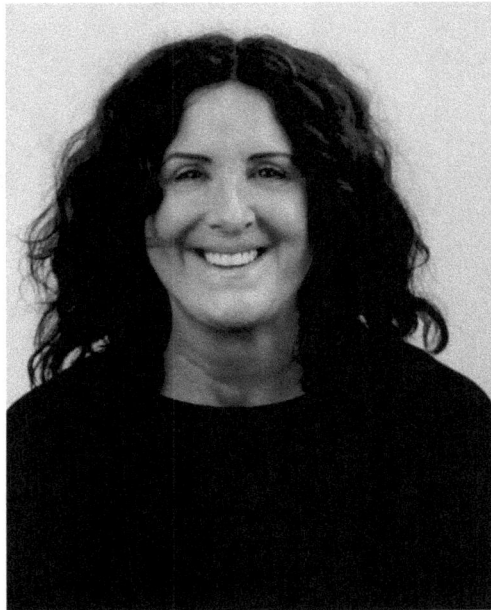

Lisa

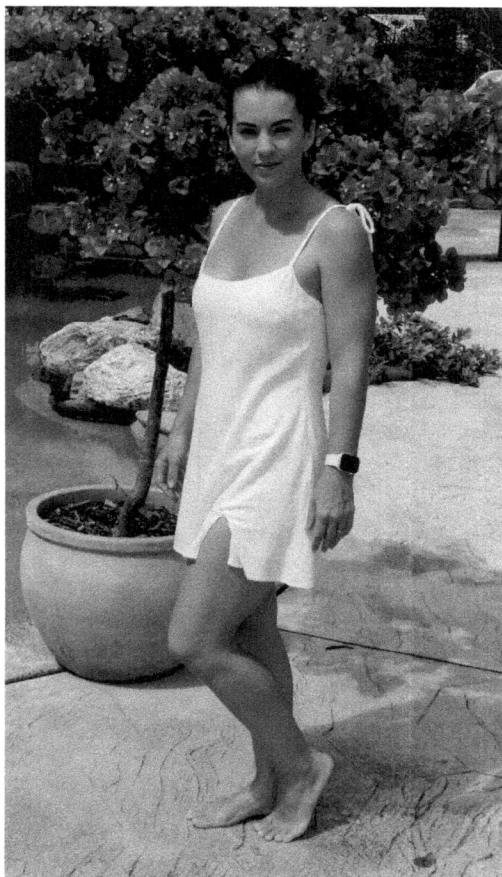

Jane

Acknowledgements

Ten very courageous women made this book possible. It's one thing to make the choice to have cosmetic surgery, but when you share your experiences, and photographs, with many others, it takes courage to another level. Not one of these women hesitated in answering any of my questions or giving permission for the use of their before and after photographs. Every one of them wanted to inspire women just like themselves. Jane, Chelsea, Julia, Rachel, Lisa, Bianca, Erica, Genevieve, Monica and Jenny, you have done just that. I am honoured to have been part of that.

My decision to self-publish was made with some trepidation. However, Kirsty Ogden and her team at Brisbane Self Publishing Service made the process seamless. The copy editing by Patrice Shaw and proofreading by Rebecca McCallion transformed the rough manuscript into something that would even please my high-school English teachers. Simone Feiler Clark at Brisbane Audiobook Production made sure that my first experience of recording a book was fun and far less daunting than I had expected. I am grateful to you all.

Operating theatre environments are quite unique. I believe patients get the best results when the staff in theatre work as a team, enjoy working with one another and are focused on the patient being safe and having the best experience possible. Every month I am privileged to work in operating theatres in Melbourne, Sydney, Rockhampton and Cairns where, in each location, the teamwork is superb. Anaesthetists, anaesthetic nurses, theatre technicians, scrub nurses, scout nurses and recovery staff are all highly skilled professionals without whom my work would not be possible. I am grateful to you all for your expertise. Special mention to Dr Peter Roessler, Dr Cliff Timmins, Dr Jeff Kallmeyer and the recently retired Dr Bill McLellan who are all exceptional anaesthetists and who I would trust to put my own family to sleep. An extra special mention to nurse Anne Miller (Millie) who is my boss in the Rockhampton theatre. She consistently goes above and beyond what is expected, making my life easier and, more importantly, making sure our patients receive the care they deserve.

Dr Mark Vucak is one of the most skilled plastic surgeons I have ever watched. He knows how to minimise his movements to provide a great result, and his ability to think outside the box to solve a surgical challenge has helped me on more than one occasion. After a hiatus from Medicine, Mark provided me with an opportunity to work with Queensland Plastic Surgery (QPS), which is something for which I will always be grateful. Without Mark or QPS, I would not have met several of the women whose stories are in this book.

Asking family members to proofread the manuscript can be risky, particularly when asking for honest feedback. My sister and brother-in-law, Denise and Darren Waterworth are becoming proofreaders extraordinaire and the suggestions from my wife's niece, Madeline Carr, were all implemented to create a manuscript that hopefully resonates with many more women.

In these days, when no plastic surgeon seems to be able to do without an Instagram account, I have been fortunate to be guided by Stephanie Allen and Ella Dumbrell at The Ardent

Collective. Stephanie edited the before and after photographs making sure essential body parts were covered, but otherwise leaving the images unaltered from when I had taken them, before and after the procedures.

Working in four different cities, spread over almost 3,000 kilometres, in three different states of Australia would be impossible without my executive assistants, Jacqui Russell-Croucher (Melbourne and Sydney) and Amanda Jackson (Cairns and Rockhampton). Both of them, mothers themselves, never cease to amaze me. They listen to our patients, are available to them 24/7 and develop personal relationships with them so that every patient knows she is respected, cared for and safe. Jac and Mandy, life is sweeter and so much more fun, knowing that we are working together, making a difference in many women's lives.

I'm sure our children, Bek, Tim, Mike and Indi roll their eyes on the first of every month when I post on our WhatsApp group, sometimes very early in the morning, to share 'pinch and a punch for the first of the month' and to let them know that I love them. Yet we are so very proud of them as they are all genuine, smart, capable and caring individuals.

Those who know my wife, Kim, would agree she is unique. When God brought her into being, I can imagine Him or Her smiling, knowing that there would be few others like her … ever. Some women are wise, some women are intelligent, some women are trustworthy, some women are beautiful. For a woman to combine all four, in such abundance, is a rarity. To be married to Kim for life is a priceless gift I treasure, and I know from the depths of my being that I am a very, very fortunate man. (Kim has just read this. She tells me she needs to go to hospital immediately because her eyes have rolled so far back into her head, they may never come out!)

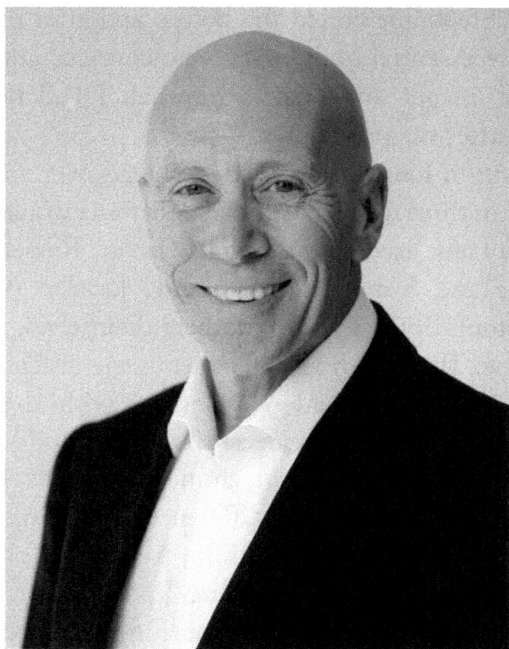

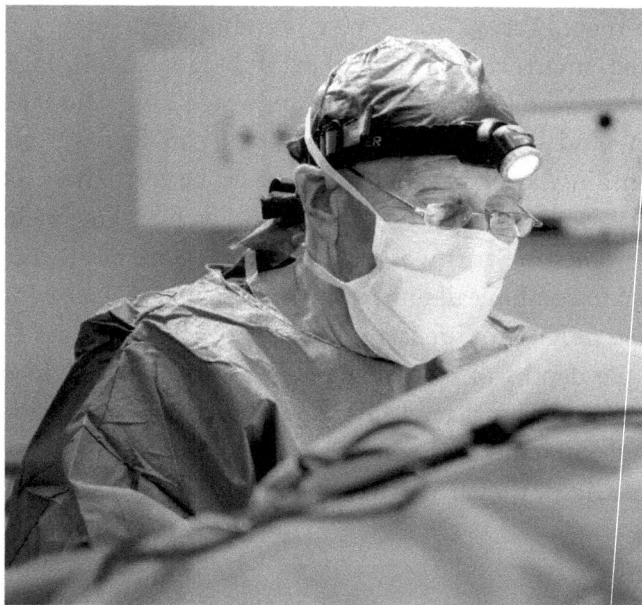

About the Author

Malcolm Linsell decided to become a doctor at the age of six. Then, following an operation on his hand at the age of thirteen, his surgeon inspired him to become a plastic surgeon. Now, after being in practice for almost thirty years, Malcolm loves making a difference in people's lives. Two to three times every week, he travels between his practices in Sydney, Melbourne, Rockhampton and Cairns in Australia. Despite the travel, every one of his patients knows he is personally available for them to contact him, twenty-four hours a day, seven days a week.

Malcolm lives in Sydney with his wife, Dr Kim Carr. An AFL fan and ever the optimist, he is anticipating his beloved St Kilda winning at least one premiership over the next few years.